THE GUIDE TO

THE HANDLING
OF PATIENTS

Third Edition

Illustrations by **Don Charlesworth,** NDD

First published 1981
Second edition 1987
Third edition 1992
   Reprinted January 1993 with amendments largely in Chapter 2

Published by National Back Pain Association 31-33 Park Road, Teddington,
Middlesex, TW11 OAB Telephone: 081-977-5474 Fax: 081-943-5318

Design by REDESIGN, Jute Lane, Enfield. Tel: 081-805 9585

Printed by Image Publicity, London 081-741 1138

A catalogue record for this publication is available from the British Library.
ISBN 0 9507726 5 8

THE GUIDE TO

THE HANDLING OF PATIENTS

E.N. Corlett, PhD, DSc, FEng, FIEE, FIMechE, ABPsS, FErgS
Scientific Adviser: Institute for Occupational Ergonomics,
University of Nottingham

P.V. Lloyd, RGN, OHNC
Adviser in Occupational Health Nursing: Royal College of
Nursing

Christine Tarling, SROT
Lifting and Handling Co-ordinator: North Tyneside Health
Care

J.D.G. Troup, PhD, DSc(Med), MRCS, LRCP, M(FOM)RCP, FErgS
Honorary Senior Research Fellow: Department of
Orthopaedic Surgery University of Aberdeen

Brenda Wright, MA, RGN, QN, RCNT
Handling Adviser; formerly Clinical Teacher,
Canterbury and Thanet Health Authority

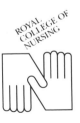

National Back Pain Association
in collaboration with the Royal College of Nursing

Contents

Foreword

As Minister of State for Health, I welcome the third edition of this guide which has been prepared by the National Back Pain Association in collaboration with the Royal College of Nursing.

Each year some 60 million working days are lost because of back pain and NHS treatment for sufferers is estimated to cost £350 million. Back pain is a major occupational hazard for nurses and other NHS staff who need to handle patients.

This publication provides an essential stimulus and shows the way forward in how to assess each handling problem in terms of the needs of the patient and disabled person; how to encourage handlers to plan and prepare the handling environment and how to choose the safest and most appropriate handling technique. It offers a unique approach to education and training combining basic ergonomics with the process of decision-making and with practical instruction in handling skills.

The NBPA are to be commended for their contribution to this field of health education.

Dr Brian Mawhinney

Minister for Health

October 1992

Acknowledgements

The acknowledgements from the first two editions of this guide are reproduced in this edition. They serve as a reminder of how much encouragement and advice has been received over the years. Without their help we would have been unable to uphold our claim that each edition has embodied the teaching that was, and is, current in the nursing, paramedical, medical, ergonomic and other scientific disciplines.

Our indebtedness now is to all members, past and present, of the RCN Advisory Panel on Back Pain; to members of 'Back Exchange' whose detailed comments have been especially valued; as well as to the following individuals whose professional input has been greatly appreciated:

Howard R Richmond BA, Solicitor, Deputy Director of Legal Services, Royal College of Nursing who is responsible for the contents of Chapter 2 of this work; he in turn acknowledges the helpful comments of all his colleagues, but in particular David Gardiner, LLB, Solicitor; Martin Spencer MA BCL (Oxon), Barrister; Lynn Young, Community Health Adviser, RCN; and his secretary Pauline Wimpory who expertly typed and retyped various drafts.

Lesley Crozier, MCSP, DipTP, for her advice on the Neuromuscular Approach;

Dr David Sines FRCN, Chair of the RCN Society for People with a Learning Handicap, and Senior Lecturer (Mental Handicap) Department of Nursing and Health Visiting, University of Ulster for help with Chapter 17;

Wendy Green, RGN, RNT, OHNC, T Cert, ACE for her input to Chapter 8;

Gesina Tait and Danielle Holmes;

and we wish to record our debt to many of Her Majesty's Judges whose comments from the Bench on the earlier editions of this Guide have been helpful and stimulating. They have enabled us to expand on sections for which our pleas of *res ipsa loquitur* were accepted with greater magnanimity than perhaps they deserved.

We would like to thank the following authors and publishers for the use of their illustrations:
Selwyn Goldsmith and RIBA Publications Ltd
Åsa Kilbom, D Sanchez & D W Grieve and Taylor & Francis Ltd
Office for Official Publications of the European Communities.

Lastly it is with great pleasure that we record the generosity of The Colt Foundation for their financial contribution to the funding of this publication.

Acknowledgements to the Second edition

The authors would like to thank their fellow members of the RCN Advisory Panel on Back Pain in Nurses for their encouragement and support. In addition they have been actively helped and supported in the preparation of this edition by:
Sarah Andrews, SRN, Isobel Johnson, MSCP, David A. Stubbs, BEd, PhD, Caroline Osborne, BSc, SRN.

Acknowledgements to the First edition

The authors have received much encouragement and help in the preparation of this guide. They would especially like to thank:
Mr C.R. Hayne FCSP, who was originally a member of the RCN/NBPA Working Party and who has given a helping hand throughout;
Professor Emeritus R.E.M. Bowden, DSc, FRCS, Miss E.P.G. Hobson, FCSP and Miss Margaret Hollis, MBE, MCSP, DipTP whose meticulous criticisms and suggestions have proved invaluable;
Esme Birchall, MCSP, Alan C. Breen, DC, Ann Brocksom, SRN, Janet R. Carruthers, MB, BS, MSc, Iain C. Gilchrist, MB, ChB, MRCGP, DObstRCOG, Hilda Hope, SEN, DN, Roz Howarth, SROT, Meryle Hudson, BSc, SRN, Jane Hughes, MCSP, Christine O'Donoghue, MCSP, Pat Rivers, BSc, SRN, SCM, DipTN, David A. Stubbs, BEd, PhD, June Sutherland, SROT, Alison Troup, MCSP, Charles Worringham, MA, Brenda Wright, MA, SRN, QN, RCNT all of whom made suggestions which have been incorporated in the text or illustrations.
The Design Manager and staff of the Design Studios, John Player and Sons for their guidance and cooperation;
and the staff of both the Back Pain Association and the Royal College of Nursing whose support has been warmly appreciated.

We also thank the Disabled Living Foundation, William Heinemann Medical Books Ltd, Mr W Brennan and Miss C Tarling for permission to make use of some of the illustrations from "Hoists and their use" in Chapter IV of this guide.

Definitions and Usages

In this edition the persons who are physically dependent on others, and who require support or assistance for their movements and activities, whether in hospital, at home or elsewhere in the community, are increasingly referred to by a variety of names which are subject to fashion and change. For the sake of simplicity, the authors will refer to all as 'patients'. The individuals on whom the said patients depend for their movements and transfers may be nurses or carers. Both words will be used and either may be referred to as 'handlers'. In order to avoid confusion when describing handling techniques, as in previous editions, the 'patient' is invariably referred to as male and the 'handler' as female.

In this guide, the words 'lift' and 'lifting' should be taken to refer to the action of raising vertically or to actions in which vertical displacement is a dominant feature. 'Transfer' and 'transferring' refer generally to actions in which the movement is mainly horizontal though some may have a vertical component. And in most transfers, some of the weight of the patient is taken by the handler (see Chapter 9). They are, however not absolute terms: many handling techniques have come to be known as, for example, Elbow Lifts although essentially they are transfer techniques. The emphasis throughout is on the need to limit the frequency and magnitude of vertical lifting or of 'dead-lifting'.

An 'assisted transfer' is one in which the patient takes some of his own weight and contributes, to a greater or lesser degree, to the movement.

Disclaimer

In this text it has not been feasible to avoid individual names of products or manufacturers, because of their common usage. In none of these instances should the appearance of such a name be taken to be a recommendation. In most cases, alternative products or manufacturers have or will have to be considered. It is for the reader to seek for guidance: for example from the Disabled Living Foundation's Information Service.

The risks associated with lifting and handling tasks are complex and each situation must be judged on its own merits and it is unreasonable for readers simply to follow the instructions in the book without proper assessment of individual circumstances.

Neither the authors nor the publisher can accept responsibility for any consequences which might result from decisions made upon the basis of the advice given therein.

PART I.
INTRODUCTION AND RESPONSIBILITY FOR ACTION

Chapter 1
Introduction

A leading article in *The Lancet* (1965), entitled 'The Nurse's Load', began with these words:

"The adult human form is an awkward burden to lift or carry. Weighing up to 100 kg. or more, it has no handles, it is not rigid, and it is liable to severe damage if mishandled or dropped. In bed a patient is placed inconveniently for lifting, and the placing of a load in such a situation would be tolerated by few industrial workers."

It went on to discuss the problems of moving and supporting patients in hospital and the community, together with the need for adequate training. It ended with these words:

"There is clearly much that can and should be done, since nursing stresses seem likely to increase as the population ages and the shortage of nurses continues. As urgent necessities the Ministry of Health might promote more ergonomic research, inquire closely into the physical requirements of the nurse's day, and ensure a wider dissemination of knowledge of lifting methods."

This message, a quarter of a century later, remains as urgent today.

It has been suggested that with the increasing emphasis on safety and the avoidance of litigation, the nursing profession is in danger of losing sight of first principles and of forgetting the needs of the patient. But it is the firm belief of the authors that greater skill in handling, the better use of handling equipment and improvement of the handling environment can only improve the patient's lot. The aim is to give the patient more control over his own activities and improve his chances of rehabilitation. Assessment of the patient is the starting point in the nursing process. It is essential to the plans that govern the patients' movements and rehabilitation. Assessment of the patient is also the starting point for the application of ergonomics to health care.

The 1st and 2nd Editions of this Guide stressed the need for ergonomics as the primary approach to the prevention of injuries and to a reduction in the physical stresses imposed on nurses; and the sug-gestions quoted above were echoed in the recommendations with which both editions concluded. But their emphasis was on the practical aspects of patient-handling: on the condemnation of unsafe lifting practices and on the need for practical instruction in the skill required for the easier and safer methods. These editions met a need and reached a wide audience. Some 30,000 copies have been bought and they have become recognised as 'codes of practice'.

The Guide, thus far, has been successful. Certainly in the experience of the authors, great improvements have been seen. The safer and better techniques have had a warm welcome. But its message has not been disseminated as widely as was hoped. The old, unsafe techniques that transgress the basic rules of lifting are still, in some places, condoned. Indeed, some are still being taught. Recommendation 6 in *The Lifting of Patients in the Health Services* from the Health Services Advisory Committee, published by HMSO in 1984:

"A positive policy on education and training in the handling of patients should be adopted and implemented by each employing authority and one person should be identified as responsible for co-ordinating all education and training in patient-handling."

has been less than faithfully observed. The principal failure has been to concentrate the policy for education and training on the recruits and learners; while senior staff and management remain immune and, often, ignorant. Thus old, unsafe, practices persist. Such employing authorities are at risk in two ways. First they will lose their nursing or caring staff because of injuries that might have been foreseen and prevented. Secondly, they face a growing threat from personal injuries litigation. But that is not all. The implementation of the EC Directive (90/269/EEC) on the minimum health and safety requirements for handling heavy loads where there is a risk of back injury for workers demands the transformation of an employer's policy. It will not be enough to rely on training of recruits to nursing and caring staff and on the practical instruction in patient-handling techniques alone. The emphasis will be on the avoidance of lifting: hence the need for more rigorous systems of assessment and the application of ergonomics. Clear warnings on the need to avoid vertical 'dead-lifting' and on the risks of attempting to lift patients and disabled people bodily without mechanical assistance were issued in the 1st and 2nd editions of the Guide. Now they are about to become mandatory. Moreover the Manual Handling Operations Regulations (1992) propose the guideline figure, as a maximum for lifting by one person, of 55 lb (25 kg). The practical implication is that when two people are required to lift or carry a disabled person the maximum is 50 kg or 112 lb. Any patient weighing 112 lb (50 kg) or more must therefore be deemed to be 'heavy' and alternatives to manual lifting must be considered.

Training in patient-handling is therefore not enough. No amount of practical skill will safeguard the nurse or carer from lifting environments or systems of work that are unsafe. In this edition, the emphasis is more directly ergonomic. It is chosen advisedly, for it is a general truth that ergonomic intervention should be cost-effective.

The starting point in the application of ergonomics to patient-handling is the patient or disabled person, his individual needs and the expectations that can reasonably be foreseen and realised. All too often, a patient is lifted or moved in obedience to a fixed routine without a thought to that individual's capacity to manage alone or with some assistance. If patients slip repeatedly down the bed, their need is not to be lifted repeatedly up the bed but for a means to stop them from sliding down and to permit them to adjust their posture at will. A little elementary ingenuity to save a lot of unnecessary exertion. Similarly, there are thousands of people in hospital and in the community who are unsteady and liable to fall. Instead of nurses and carers being put at risk by attempting to save them from falling or, indeed, by lifting them manually from the floor; the solution may be to teach patients how to fall safely – a routine matter in physiotherapy – and how to get to their feet again with minimal help. For a heavy patient in intensive care, mechanical equipment would be obligatory: at least until rehabilitation can begin.

At a practical level, the implementation of an ergonomics based policy for patient-handling is quite simple: through the medium of the Care Plan. Care Plans also provide the vehicle for the assessment of manual handling tasks which is the major requirement in the EC Directive (90/269/EEC: adopted 29 May 1990, in force from 31st December 1992).

Chapter 2
Legal and Professional Responsibilities

(by H R Richmond BA, Solicitor, Deputy Director of Legal Services, Royal College of Nursing)

Introduction

The Law, as it relates to the lifting and handling of patients, has two principal objectives, accident prevention and compensation for the injured lifter.

Accident prevention is regulated by statute, principally in the form of the Health and Safety at Work etc. Act 1974 (HSWA74). Compensation for injury to the lifter is provided for mainly by the Common Law, that is, law contained in previous decisions of the Courts which assume the force of binding or persuasive precedent.

Accident Prevention by Statute

Section 2(1), HSWA74 imposes a duty on every employer ". . . to ensure, so far as is reasonably practicable, the health, safety, and welfare at work of all his employees". The scope of the duty is further clarified in Section 2(2) to include in particular, but only so far as is reasonably practicable:

(a)   The provision and maintenance of plant and work systems, that are safe and without health risks;

(b)   Arrangements for ensuring safety and absence of health risks in the use, handling, storage and transport of articles and substances;

(c)   Provision of information, instruction, training and supervision necessary to ensure health and safety;

(d)   Maintenance of any place of work under the employer's control, and all means of access and egress from it in a condition that is safe and without health risks;

(e)   Provision and maintenance of a working environment that is safe and without risks to health and adequate as regards facilities and arrangements for welfare at work.

With regard to lifting and handling patients, the most relevant duties are contained in paragraphs (a), equipment and systems of work and (c), instruction and training, but all apply to some extent. The duty is not an absolute one. It is qualified by the important words 'so far as is reasonably practicable'. An employer needs to comply with this duty only if the cost of providing, say, equipment or training is not grossly disproportionate to the benefit. Were the benefit to be minimal and the cost substantial, an employer might be relieved of complying with a duty (Edwards – v – National Coal Board)*.

Under Section 7, HSWA74 the employee is under a corresponding duty to take reasonable care for his or her own health and safety and those who may be affected by his or her acts or omissions, and to co-operate with the employer in performing its duties under the Act.

Where it is reasonably practicable to comply with one of these duties and the employer fails to do so, enforcement action can be taken by the Health and Safety Executive (HSE). HSE Inspectors have a right of entry to conduct inspections and a power to serve Improvement Notices specifying particulars of the breach of health and safety law contravened and specifying a time within which the breach should be remedied. An example might be to require provision of suitable lifting equipment in an orthopaedic ward with heavy, highly dependent patients, where there is no hoist available. An HSE Inspector has the additional power to serve a Prohibition Notice preventing activities being carried out if there is a risk of serious personal injury. Failure to comply with Improvement or Prohibition Notices, or commission of a breach of the general duties in Section 2(2)(a) – (e) in, or any regulations made under, HSWA74 can give rise to a criminal prosecution. On conviction in the Crown Court the maximum penalties in the most serious cases are two years imprisonment and an unlimited fine. In the Magistrates Court, where the vast majority of cases are heard, the maximum fine is £20,000, and where the conviction relates to failure to comply with

* [1949] 1 All E.R. 743

Prohibition or Improvement Notices, up to six months imprisonment.* Where an offence is committed by a corporate body, senior managers or directors can also be made individually liable where the offence was committed with the consent or connivance of that manager or attributable to that manager's neglect.

Accident Prevention by Regulation and Guidance

The HSWA74 is a general enabling Act which allows the Secretary of State to make regulations and for the Health and Safety Commission (HSC) to issue codes of practice and guidance notes. The Manual Handling Operations Regulations 1992 (MHO Regs 92) govern the lifting and handling of patients in the workplace. To a lesser extent the Management of Health and Safety at Work Regulations 1992 (M of HSW Regs 92), the Provision and Use of Work Equipment Regulations 1992 and the Workplace (Health, Safety and Welfare) Regulations 1992 also apply. These Regulations aim to translate into domestic law the UK's obligations under various European Community Directives relevant to Health and Safety law. These Directives are discussed more fully later in this Chapter. As with accident prevention by statute, a breach of any provision in these regulations can ultimately lead to a prosecution being brought by HSE.

Regulation 3(1) of the M of HSW Regs 92 requires employers to make a suitable and sufficient assessment of all the risks to the health and safety of their employees while at work. Where this general assessment indicates the possibility of risks to employees from the manual handling of loads the provisions of Regulation 4 of the MHO Regs 92 come into play. The employer is required to follow a three stage procedure: first, to avoid manual handling operations involving a risk of injury, so far as is reasonably practicable; second, where such hazardous manual handling operations cannot with reasonable practicability be avoided, to make suitable and sufficient assessment of such operations having regard to certain factors involving the task, the load, the working environment, and the individual capabilities of the lifters almost identical to the reference factors set out in Table 1 on page 22; thirdly and finally, informed by the assessment the employer must take appropriate steps to reduce the risk of injury to the lowest level reasonably practicable. This assessment must be kept up to date, and the employee must be given a general indication, and where reasonably practicable, precise information on the weight of the load. In general, the assessment should be recorded and be readily available.

The MHO Regs 92 are accompanied by HSE guidance on the subject. This guidance note does not

have the force of law. Nevertheless HSE Inspectors can take it into account when considering whether there is compliance with the MHO Regs. For instance Appendix I, paragraph 10 of the guidance note contains a diagram of guideline weight figures. Although these are stressed not to be weight or force limits, it is arguable that these guideline figures indicate the threshold beyond which there is a risk of the employee being injured. A failure on the part of an employer to carry out an assessment of manual handling operations prior to these guideline figures being exceeded might well be evidence of a breach of the MHO Regs 92 but it would be for a Court to decide the issue. Further, paragraph 42 of the guidance note indicates that an assessment made at the last minute is unlikely to be suitable and sufficient as required by the Regulations; employers must look in a considered way at the whole range of manual handling operations required of employees. Generic assessments drawing together common threads from a range of broadly similar operations are considered acceptable. The M of HSW Regs 92 are accompanied by an Approved Code of Practice (ACoP). In any prosecution where it is proved that there is a failure to observe a relevant provision in an ACoP, the burden of proof falls on the Defendant to show that regulations are satisfied in some way, other than by observing the ACoP.

The Health Services Advisory Committee to the Health and Safety Commission published guidance entitled *The Lifting of Patients in the Health Services* in 1984 and this has now been updated in its *Guidance on manual handling of loads in the Health Services* 1992. This guidance can also be taken into account by a Court but only as assistance in considering whether there is evidence of breach. A suitable analogy might be with the Highway Code. A breach of the Highway Code might well be evidence of an offence under the Road Traffic Acts or of negligence in civil law but by no means conclusively so.

There is also guidance of an unofficial nature; this volume itself, for instance; or the Code of Practice for the Handling of Patients, first issued by the Royal College of Nursing in 1982 and now updated. The status of these documents is that of expert opinion. Such opinion may well be very persuasive in that it represents the consensus of foremost experts in the field, and in the case of the Code of Practice, endorsed by the leading professional nursing organisation in the UK. However, such opinion is no more than potentially very persuasive on any aspect until approved by a Court, and it would be open to any Defendant in Court proceedings to bring expert evidence to the contrary. Furthermore, these documents are not admissible in court proceedings on their own; they have to be drawn on and supported by an expert witness in each case. This point is discussed in more detail in the following section on compensation.

---

* Section 4 Offshore Safety Act 1992.

Compensation

Section 47 HSWA74 expressly states that breach of the general duties in Section 2(2)(a) – (e) HSWA74 does not give rise to civil liability, that is, breach of these general duties does not entitle an employee injured in a lifting and handling accident to compensation. However, this is a distinction without a difference in practice, since the Common Law places equivalent duties on the employer to take reasonable care for the safety of its employees and so to carry out its operations as not to subject employees to unnecessary risk. This is a personal responsibility which cannot be delegated.

The modern authority for the employer's duty is set out in a House of Lords case (Wilsons and Clyde Coal Ltd – v – English**) which requires that all employers provide and maintain, so far as is reasonable:

(a) A safe place of work with safe means of access and egress;

(b) safe appliances, equipment, and plant for doing work;

(c) a safe system for doing work;

(d) competent and safety conscious personnel.

In addition, the employer is responsible for the negligence of its employees even if the employer is not itself at fault. This is known as Vicarious Liability, a legal principle which often causes confusion to lay people. It is discussed further under Problem Areas later in this Chapter.

Claims for compensation for injury, usually back injury, arising from the lifting and handling of patients are most often pursued on the basis of the employer's failure to provide a safe system of work, although a failure to provide equipment, a safe place of work, or competent fellow personnel can also be factors. The Plaintiff has to prove that the employer has breached its duty in one of the above respects and that that breach of duty caused the injury. Each case is argued on its particular merits and expert evidence is required to prove, first, what reasonably safe system of work could have avoided the accident, and secondly, in what respects the employer fell short of that duty in the particular case before the Court.

Previous editions of The Handling of Patients have assisted Courts to decide on the standard to be attained. For instance, in the case of Edwards – v – Waltham Forest Health Authority (1989)* Mr Justice Potts stated:

"I have reached the conclusion that the standards set out in page 5 of The Handling of Patients, A Guide for Nurse Managers and the measures to be adopted on bath transfers as described at page 35 [which provides that lifting

a patient manually out of a bath should only be necessary in an emergency if a patient is taken ill or helpless and under no other circumstances] were well known in the nursing profession in April 1982. I am also satisfied upon the evidence that I have heard that those standards and measures were entirely proper and were the standards and measures that could and should have been adopted by all competent employers for their employees. I have to say that I am surprised that in this case, on the evidence, no responsible person at [the] hospital seems to have applied his or her mind to what is set out in this volume, and in particular to those parts mentioned".

It should not be assumed that The Handling of Patients sets the standard to be achieved in all circumstances. Although it embodies the opinion of several foremost experts in the field, its application to the facts of any particular case must be proved by an expert witness; a Defendant could bring other experts to argue that in any particular set of circumstances the advice given was not appropriate or reasonable.

The landmark case in the field is that of Williams – v – Gwent Health Authority (1982)*** where the Defendant was held to be liable for having an unsafe system of work in allowing the Drag Lift to be used. Since that time Plaintiffs have recovered compensation where unsafe systems have been found in the use of the Orthodox Lift (Moore – v – Norfolk Health Authority, 1982)*, in respect of falling patients, (Bayley – v – Bloomsbury Health Authority, 1987)* and in respect of a District Nurse lifting a patient on her own (Hammond – v – Cornwall and Isles of Scilly Health Authority, 1986) and in respect of the use of The Australian Lift on a heavy patient where a hoist should have been used (Munro – v – Plymouth Health Authority 1991*). In addition, a health authority has been found vicariously liable where a co-lifter failed to lift on the count of three, injuring the lifter taking the lead (Page – v – Enfield and Haringey Health Authority, 1985*). Staff shortages provide a consistent backcloth to lifting accidents but courts are reluctant to find breach of duty on this ground alone (Stewart – v – Highland Health Board 1987*).

As has been said, breach of the general duties in section 2 (2) (a) – (e) HSWA74 do not give rise to civil liability. However, breaches of provisions in regulations made under HSWA74 can give rise to civil liability for what is called breach of statutory duty unless the regulations provide otherwise. Regulation 15 of the M of HSW Regs 92 states that a breach of duty imposed by those regulations does not confer a right of any action in any civil proceedings (although this may not prevent the duties set out in the parent Framework Directive 89/391/EEC being directly effective for which we see the section headed 1992 Developments below). There is no such exclusion in the MHO Regs 92. This means that a breach of any duty in Regulation 4 setting out the assessment procedure can be invoked in a civil claim. In this context it should be

* Unreported
** [1938] A.C. 57.
*** [1983] C.L.Y. 255.

noted that the duty to carry out an assessment where there is a risk of injury is almost absolute, that is to say, there will be no defence to a failure to carry out an assessment save perhaps to plead that there was no risk of injury at all. The application of the findings of the assessment are subject to the test of 'reasonable practicability'. The employer will only be relieved of liability if it can show that the cost of putting into effect the findings of the assessment would be grossly disproportionate to the benefit. Further, such cost benefit calculations must have been made prior to the incident giving rise to the claim. In principle, therefore, the MHO Regs should make it easier for a Plaintiff to prove breach of duty.

As well as proving the breach of duty itself, the Plaintiff has to prove, with the assistance of expert medical evidence, that the breach of duty caused the injury sustained. This is by no means straight forward, since lifters can often be shown to have vulnerable backs, either resulting from naturally occurring degenerative changes, or from previous back injuries, or from the effects of cumulative strain from regular heavy lifting. It is difficult to obtain the evidence necessary to pursue a claim based on cumulative strain alone. In most cases one is considering the injury caused by a particular lifting incident and the effect that incident may have in aggravating and/or accelerating existing injury, albeit symptom free, until that incident occurred. Where pre-existing vulnerability is proved to exist, compensation can be significantly reduced.

Although the Plaintiff in a civil claim has to prove negligence, namely that the breach of duty caused the injury, this is not an end in itself; it is only a means to an end, which is compensation. The aim of financial compensation is to put the Plaintiff back into the position she would have been in if the accident had not happened. Where loss of earnings and extra expense are incurred, the arithmetic at least can be fairly straightforward. Lawyers call these Special Damages. Financial compensation for pain and suffering, restricted lifestyle, or a destroyed career whose path can only be guessed at, are more difficult and controversial. The trial judge has some discretion in assessing these so called General Damages within a framework of principles set down in previously decided cases.

Awards for pain and suffering and loss of amenity made by English Courts are considered by many to be too low. Back injuries attract awards in the range of £1,000 to £20,000 depending on the degree of severity. However, where a lifter's career is destroyed by the accident, awards can be greatly boosted by compensation for past and future loss of earnings and recent awards have fallen in the range £150,000 – £205,000. Thus, although compensation claims are not intended to be punitive, the amounts which can be ordered to be paid are many orders of magnitude greater than any fines which might be levied under the HSWA74 and in this regard com-

pensation claims could be considered to have an indirect deterrent effect. The value of potential claims should certainly form part of the risk benefit calculation which might lead employers to decide in favour of allocating more resources in carrying out their duties.

Defendants routinely allege that Plaintiffs are partly to blame for the accident in question; this is called contributory negligence. A finding of contributory negligence does not defeat the claim, it merely serves to reduce the compensation. For example a Plaintiff found to be twenty-five per cent to blame would have her compensation reduced by twenty-five per cent. Experience to date shows that courts have been reluctant to make such findings in nurse lifting cases.

Although emphasis has been placed on compensation which can be recovered through bringing a civil action, it must be mentioned that compensation is available from other sources where an employee is incapable of working through sickness or accident. There may be an entitlement to sick pay from the employer, but only if provided for in the contract of employment. Employers also administer the Statutory Sick Pay Scheme which provides benefits for the first 28 weeks of sickness. Beyond that, Sickness/ Invalidity Benefit may be available from the Department of Social Security. Of particular relevance is the Industrial Injuries Scheme which provides Disablement Benefit to compensate those who have suffered disablement from a loss of physical or mental faculty caused by an industrial accident. However, benefit is only payable where the loss of faculty amounts to 14% or more. Of particular interest to National Health Service employees is the NHS Injury Benefits Scheme which should be better known than it is. Benefit is payable to all NHS employees regardless of length of employment who suffer an injury because of NHS employment. There are separate schemes for those absent temporarily through injury and those whose employment is terminated. The aim is to compensate for reduction of earning ability caused by the injury and, depending on length of service and degree of reduction in earning ability, benefits can be awarded up to a maximum of 85% of pre-injury pay, together with entitlement to a lump sum on termination of employment. Where compensation is recovered in a civil action, NHS Injury Benefit payments have to be repaid or adjusted. In this respect they can be considered to be payments on account of compensation although no fault need be proved.

With regard to Social Security Benefits, all payments made to injured employees for accidents after 1 January 1989 must be repaid by the employer to the DSS where compensation is agreed or ordered to be paid in excess of £2,500. This provision, subject to much criticism, has had adverse effects on Plaintiffs. However, there are indirect deterrent effects on employers, who now bear some of the costs of supporting injured employees previously borne by the tax payer.

Employment and Professional Conduct

There are two other minor aspects to the law which must be mentioned for completeness. First, an employee owes a duty to the employer to obey reasonable and lawful instructions and to act with reasonable care and skill. Thus a failure to perform as trained or instructed could render the employee liable to disciplinary proceedings.

Further, some professional persons involved in lifting and handling are subject to codes of conduct. For instance, a nurse who refused to carry out what she considered was an unsafe lift was referred to the United Kingdom Central Council Professional Conduct Committee but was found not guilty of conduct unbefitting a nurse (UKCC – v – Lalis Lilian Grant, *Nursing Standard* 18/2/89)*.

Clause 13 of the 3rd edition (June 1992) of the Code of Professional Conduct for the Nurse, Midwife and Health Visitor states:

"Report to an appropriate person or authority where it appears that the health or safety of colleagues is at risk, as such circumstances may compromise standards of care and practice."

It is therefore conceivable that a senior nurse with responsibility for lifting and handling standards of safety could be rendered accountable to the nursing professional body as well as to the Court. Further, there is a professional duty on all nurses to report their concerns.

1992 Developments

Important changes in the health and safety field have been brought about as a result of the completion of the single market in the European Community (EC) on 31 December 1992.

The aim of the legislation is to harmonise health and safety standards throughout the EC such that undertakings operating in a country which might otherwise have lower health and safety standards and therefore lower costs, do not have an unfair competitive advantage. This process is described in the jargon as the creation of a 'level playing field'.

Authority for the legislation arises principally from Article 118a of the Treaty of Rome 1957 (amended by the Single European Act 1987) which has the objective of harmonising health and safety standards in the EC and encouraging and maintaining improvements in those standards. Article 100a which aims to remove technical barriers to trade is also relevant. The main instrument by which these aims are translated into domestic law is through the Directive. A Directive places obligations on a member state as to the result to be achieved by domestic legislation,

---

* Unreported

but leaves open to each state the form and method of implementation as long as this is done within a stated time limit. Problems have arisen where Directives have not been complied with either at all, or insufficiently.

Recent decisions of the European Court, and of the UK House of Lords have had the effect of upgrading the status and force of EC Directives. The arguments are complex and will doubtless be litigated over the next few years. However, there is a significant force of legal opinion behind the following propositions in respect of the force and effect of Directives namely:

1. that where Directives are sufficiently clear and precise, unconditional, and leave no room for discretion in implementation; that they are binding on EC members' National Courts, in relation to civil claims at least, whether or not the Plaintiff relies on them;

2. that they must be enforced by National Courts against all classes of Defendant whether in the public or private sector;

3. that breach of provisions in Directives relating to Health and Safety can constitute breaches of duty in English common law negligence or breach of statutory duty even from the date of the Directive itself and regardless of implementation in domestic law, because National Courts are now compelled to interpret existing domestic law in the light of Directives;

4. that in interpreting EC law National Courts must adopt the 'purposive' approach of the continental civil law tradition, to be contrasted with the much narrower 'textual' approach of the English common law stressing as it does the meaning of words;

5. that if the domestic law falls short of the requirements of any Directive the National Court must interpret the domestic law in the light of the wording of the Directive and if necessary 're-write' it to rectify the omission; and

6. that an individual who has been harmed as a result of the failure of a member state to take all necessary steps to achieve the result required by a Directive can, subject to certain conditions, sue the member state for compensation.

In the light of these principles it is therefore best to concentrate on the provisions of the relevant Directives themselves, rather than the regulations made under the HSWA74 referred to above, as the text of the Directive is likely to prevail where there is any inconsistency with the wording in the regulation. In the lifting and handling field these are principally the Council Directive of 12 June 1989 (89/391/EEC) on the introduction of measures to encourage improvements in the safety and health of workers at work, the so called Framework Directive intended to be implemented by the M of HSW Regs 92, and the Council Directive of 29 May 1990 (90/269/EEC) on the minimum health and safety requirements for the manual handling of loads where there is a risk particularly of back injury to workers, the Manual Handling of Loads Directive intended to be implemented by the MHO Regs 92.

The Manual Handling of Loads Directive is subsidiary to the Framework Directive and should be interpreted in the light of it. Article 5.1 of the Framework Directive provides that:

> "The employer shall have a duty to ensure the safety and health of workers in every aspect related to the work".

Article 6.1 and 6.2 provide:

"1. Within the context of his responsibilities the employer shall take measures necessary for the safety and health protection of workers, including prevention of occupational risks and provision of information and training, as well as provision of the necessary organisation and means. The employer shall be alert to the need to adjust these measures to take account of changing circumstances and aim to improve existing situations.

2. The employer shall implement the measures referred to . . . [above] . . . on the basis of the following general principles on prevention:

     (a) avoiding risks;

     (b) evaluating the risks which cannot be avoided;

     (c) combating the risks at source;

     (d) adapting the work to the individual, especially as regards the design of work places, the choice of work equipment and the choice of working and production methods, with a view, in particular, to alleviating monotonous work and work at a predetermined work-rate and to reducing their effect on health;

     (e) adapting to technical progress;

     (f) replacing the dangerous by the non-dangerous or the less dangerous;

     (g) developing a coherent overall prevention policy which covers technology, organization of work, working conditions, social relationships and the influence of factors related to the working environment;

     (h) giving collective protective measures priority over individual protective measures;

     (i) giving appropriate instructions to the workers."

The above general obligations do not contain the limitation familiar from the HSWA to exercise duties "so far as is reasonably practicable" or to take only "reasonable" care as required by common law. The only limitation permitted under the Framework Directive is in Article 5.4 which provides:

> "This Directive shall not restrict the option of member states to provide for the exclusion or the limitation of the employer's responsibility where occurrences are due to unusual and unforeseeable circumstances, beyond the employer's control, or to exceptional events, the consequences of which could not have been avoided despite the exercise of all due care."

It will certainly be argued that the effect of the Framework Directive is to impose a higher duty on employers more near to that of 'practicability' rather than 'reasonable practicability'. In essence, this means that a duty must be performed if it is capable of performance in the technical sense, economic considerations not being relevant.

As indicated above the M of HSW Regs 92 cannot be invoked in support of a civil compensation claim. Further, they relegate the obligations in article 6.2 (a) – (i) to paragraph 27 of the accompanying Approved Code of Practice. Both devices arguably amount to an insufficient implementation of the Framework Directive.

The Manual Handling of Loads Directive, which must be read in the light of the Framework Directive, provides in Articles 3 and 4:

"3.1 The employer shall take appropriate organisational measures, or shall use the appropriate means, in particular mechanical equipment, in order to avoid the need for the manual handling of loads by workers.

3.2 Where the need for the manual handling of loads by workers cannot be avoided the employer shall take the appropriate organisational measures, use the appropriate means, or provide workers with such means in order to reduce the risk involved in the manual handling of such loads, having regard to . . . [various reference factors set out in an annex relating to the characteristics of the load, the physical effort required, the characteristics of the working environment, and the requirements of the activity which is reproduced in full in Table 1 on page 22 below].

4 Wherever the need for manual handling of loads by workers cannot be avoided, the employer shall organise workstations in such a way as to make such handling as safe and healthy as possible and:

     (a) Assess in advance if possible, the health and safety conditions of the type of work involved, and in particular examine the characteristics of loads taking account of . . . [the reference factors in the annex referred to above].

(b) Take care to avoid or reduce the risk particularly of back injury to workers, by taking appropriate measures, considering in particular the characteristics of the working environment and the requirements of the activity, taking account of . . . [the reference factors in the annex referred to above]".

Again the extent of the duty which Article 3.1 imposes on employers is arguably higher than the standard of 'reasonable practicability' required by the MHO Regs 92. However, paragraph 108 of the guidance note to the MHO Regs 92 itself emphasises the ergonomic approach advocated by previous editions of this publication. Further, the HSE emphasises that the costs of mechanising lifting procedures, although expensive, will lead to productivity gains and to cost savings from reducing injury. It is therefore likely that regardless of whether the Framework and Manual Handling of Loads Directives conflict with the M of HSW Regs 92 and/or the MHO Regs 92, employers will be required to provide hoists and/or other appropriate equipment in lifting patients heavier than the guideline figures and that a failure to do so may lead to legal consequences both as regards regulation and as regards compensation.

The key change fully implemented in the MHO Regs 92 is the requirement of assessment prior to lifting or handling any patients where the lifting or handling manoeuvre is such as to carry a risk of injury which cannot otherwise be avoided. Of particular relevance in the ward situation is Article 6.1.2(d) of the Framework Directive quoted above relating to the rate of work which might have significant implications for ward routines.

Equipment

Since legal developments in the field are likely to lead to increased use of equipment and other aids, it is appropriate to mention the employer's duties as regards work equipment. As has been stated, both the common law duty and the general duty under the Health and Safety at Work Act is similar, namely, to provide and maintain work equipment in so far as is reasonably practicable. The employer can seek to ensure proper maintenance of and training for the use of equipment, but may not be able to avoid a hidden defect in its manufacture. However, where an employee sustains personal injury because of a defect in equipment provided by the employer, and the defect is the fault of another party, for example the manufacturer or maintenance contractor, the injury is still deemed to be attributable to the fault of the employer [Employers Liability (Defective Equipment) Act 1969]. In other words, the employer cannot defend a claim of negligence even though entirely blameless. The employer may have a claim against the third party be it manufacturer or contractor but is itself primarily responsible for compensating the injured employee if the third party is proved or admitted to be negligent.

Alternatively, the injured employee may be able to claim compensation under Part I of the Consumer Protection Act 1987. A product is "defective" if the safety of the product is "not such as persons generally are entitled to expect". There is an advantage here in that fault need not be shown. However, the employee can only claim against the employer if the manufacturer cannot be identified.

Work equipment is further regulated under an EC Directive of 30 November 1989 concerning the minimum health and safety requirements for the use of work equipment by workers (89/655/EEC). This obliges employers to take the measures necessary to ensure either that work equipment can be used without risk to safety, or, if there is a risk, to minimise such risk. This is to be achieved by selecting new equipment after 31 December 1992 which complies with certain minimum standards set out in an annex to the Directive, and in relation to existing equipment, to ensure that it complies with such minimum standards by 31 December 1996 either by replacement on or before that date, or, by ensuring adequate maintenance to achieve such minimum standards throughout its further working life. Employers must take necessary measures to ensure that employees have adequate information and where appropriate, written instructions containing at the minimum the conditions of use of work equipment, foreseeable abnormal situations, and conclusions to be drawn from experience, where appropriate, in using work equipment. Such information and instruction must be comprehensible to the workers concerned. Adequate training in the use of any work equipment must be provided including training on any risks which such use may entail. Such obligations are translated into UK law in the Provision and Use of Work Equipment Regulations 1992.

Problem Areas

Concern is often expressed in three particular areas: the legal responsibilities of the lifting trainer towards the student, the duty of the employer where a member of the lifting team is not an employee but an agency worker whose training or competence is an unknown factor, and of the professionally trained lifting instructor towards the carer.

The lifting trainer owes a duty to provide proper instruction and supervision to trainees, so far as is reasonable, and the duty is greater, the more inexperienced the trainees. In the case of Beattie – v – West Dorset Health Authority (1990) the Plaintiff was injured during a training session. She and a co-trainee who was seven and a half inches taller than her were practising the use of the Cradle or Orthodox Lift. Another trainee weighing ten and a half stones acted as the patient. The Court held that the trainer was negligent in pairing the Plaintiff with a

* Unreported

totally inexperienced and significantly taller partner without instructing that partner in how to compensate for the height difference, and in failing to intervene to prevent them from practising a hazardous lift.

Where the trainer is acting in the course of employment, the employer must meet any claim by providing legal representation, satisfying any Court judgement, or paying any compensation which may be agreed between the parties. The employer's obligation stems from the doctrine of vicarious liability mentioned above. It applies regardless of whether the employer is itself negligent by, for instance, failing to fully train the trainer. The employee trainer is always wise to ensure that the precise scope of training duties is set out in writing in the contract of employment or job description. The doctrine of vicarious liability only applies to events taking place in the course of employment and not to acts committed by employees who are, in the delightful phraseology used by the Courts "off on a frolic of their own"!

Where the lifting trainer is not an employee but an independent contractor, the employer's duty to provide a safe system for training in the lifting and handling of patients, so far as is reasonable, remains. The employer can delegate performance of its duties to provide such a safe system, but never its responsibility. The employer can discharge its responsibility by taking reasonable care in the selection of independent contractors. In the future, the scope of this duty may be significantly tightened by the impact of Article 5.2 of the Framework Directive which provides that where the employer enlists competent external services or persons to comply with its obligations under the Directive, this shall not "discharge him from his responsibilities in this area".

This leads on to the situation of the agency worker contracted in to form part of a lifting and handling team. It is arguable that the employer must take reasonable steps to ensure that any outside contractor has been trained and assessed as competent in lifting and handling patients and that if it fails to do so,

it is in breach of duty to its own employees who may be injured as a result of that contractor's lifting error. However, the combined effects of Articles 5.2 and 5.4 of the Framework Directive would suggest that employers may be legally responsible for the failures of outside contractors regardless of fault in most circumstances.

The problems arising from the lifting and handling of patients in the community are far greater because the health care provider has only limited control over conditions in the patient's home, while still under an obligation to provide a reasonably safe system of work for its employees when lifting and handling patients in the home setting. One problem that can arise is where patients or relatives refuse a hoist where assessment indicates this is necessary to minimise risk of injury to the community nurse. Where all reasonable efforts have been made to achieve acceptance of such recommendations, it would be reasonable of management to inform the patient that services might have to be withdrawn.

Lifting and handling often involves securing the assistance of carers who are family members and who may often, themselves, be elderly or disabled. It can be said that the community or district nurse has a duty to teach such carers to lift safely both by assessing the carer's ability to lift, and by teaching them the principles of safe lifting and assessing their level of competence. This would apply both to manual techniques and to the use of any appropriate lifting aids which may be provided. A carer who is injured may have a claim against the provider of community care services if such training can be proved to have fallen below the standard of training which expert opinion considers a carer should receive. However, since there is no employer/employee relationship between the carer and the health care provider the claim would be made under the general law of professional negligence; as such it will face problems of foreseeability, standard of care to be expected, causation, and the reluctance of Courts to 'open the floodgates' to new categories of claims.

Chapter 3
Ergonomics and Health Care

Introduction

Ergonomics is the application of knowledge from the human and physical sciences to the creation of a match between people and their activities, the environment in which they find themselves and the equipment they operate. Although ergonomics is applicable to all human activity, it is of particular relevance in the working world. There, decisions may have to be taken or tasks pursued at a time or at speeds that are not freely chosen by the individual. The larger the organisation in which the work is done, the greater the emphasis on communication between all the individuals engaged upon it. Ergonomics, if it is to be successful, must take all these factors into account. Then, if the work is ergonomically satisfactory, the work is safe, satisfying for its operators and efficient by any standards of good management.

Ergonomics is the subject which looks at how things, jobs, environments etc. are matched to people's sizes, strengths, abilities and other human attributes. It takes the position that situations should be designed primarily for those people involved with them. It is a 'people centred' viewpoint rather than a job centred one. The consequence of good ergonomics in a workplace is more effective, healthier and less stressful work, which is a benefit to everyone.

Most jobs have just grown. Something has required doing, someone has done it and so a job is born. However, there are many cultural influences which restrict the content or characteristics of jobs. Until very recently machines were designed to do their tasks, and people had to adapt to the machines. This meant learning their particular characteristics and foibles, as well as putting up with their inadequacies. Culture restricts certain jobs to certain people, not just due to the knowledge requirement either. The common perception of 'nurse' is still that of a woman, for example.

So, if we study a task without looking at it from a person centred perspective, as well as recognising that the reasons for some things being done the way they are may be organisational or cultural conventions, then we shall miss many opportunities for improvement by allowing ourselves to be locked into the current, inappropriate frame of reference.

Notice that ergonomics is not just about forces and postures. It is about how all relevant factors influence a person's ability to perform a job. In any practical assessment, however, we recognise that everything cannot be done at once, so some selection is necessary. Here the assessment focuses on the problems of load-handling, which are major contributors to injury in the health care professions and their supporting services. Even with this focus, it would be insufficient to study only load and posture. Our start must be to identify the contributing factors and then to use this knowledge to guide our assessment and evaluation procedures.

The first question asked by an ergonomist when analysing a given task or working process is, why is this job being done? What function does it serve? Thus when ergonomics is applied to health care, the question becomes oriented towards the patient and his needs. What is being done for the patient? What is the best way of achieving it?. The questions which follow depend on the adequacy of the assessment of the patient. Answers will be needed on what the patient can prudently do for himself, on what equipment may be needed and, if the nurse or carer should take an active, physical role, what exactly is required. On the one hand, what forces may have to be exerted; and on the other, what is the physical work capacity of the nurse or carer to whom the task may fall.

When the basic ergonomic questions are put in manufacturing and service industries, it is usually possible to answer in more or less precise terms. In health care, it is less easy. The element of uncertainty is more prevalent. The 'patient' does not come in stock sizes or conditions. The physical dependence of the patient varies from infinite to nil. The medical constraints, from intravenous drips to plaster jackets, are protean. And there is the additional uncertainty of patients' behaviour. All these elements have to be considered and weighed ergonomically (McAtamney and Corlett 1992). Otherwise the task for nurse or carer remains undefined and left to the spur of the moment; and no attempt is made to create a match between the task and the nurses and carers who may be at risk.

Ergonomics is not only concerned with analysis of an existing task or process. It is essential when designing afresh for the environment in which health care is offered and when selecting the equipment. It is also applied in the form of improvement: for example, the occupational therapist applies her ergonomic skills when advising a stroke patient on how to adapt his home to give him greater independence; how to adapt the home to allow his carers to work more safely and more efficiently.

But to begin with ergonomics will often have to be applied to the recognition of difficult situations. Circumstances such as the confined spaces of a house or ambulance, or particular conditions in hospital for patient care, may make otherwise suitable equipment inadequate or, indeed, unsafe. For example, though a fixed toilet rail in a lavatory assists the ambulant patient, it may be a wholly inappropriate fitting for a lavatory that is used for wheelchair dependent patients. Thus all is grist to the ergonomic mill: the needs of the patient in all their variety; architectural considerations; the selection and design of furniture, fittings and equipment; communication; definition of the workload; and the working capacity of individual nurses and carers. If the ergonomic brief thus seems impossibly large and infinitely complex, take heart. None of these considerations go beyond the bounds of common sense and practical experience. What is needed is recognition of unsafe or awkward working practices and environments and a fresh approach to assessment. That will be the first step in ergonomics. It will also serve the requirements of the Manual Handling Operations Regulations.

Handling Loads

The handling of loads, whether human or inanimate, is a common experience in the world of health care. It is also an aspect of work to which an appreciation of ergonomics can bring solutions. We shall look at load-handling from a number of viewpoints: how the body copes with imposed loads and the effects on the handler of the surroundings and circumstances under which the load must be handled.

It is axiomatic that, if possible, lifting and handling is avoided. Do not rush to lift things or people without pausing to ask if it is necessary. A load can be left where it is; or slid; or handling equipment can be made ready. A patient can be encouraged to shift for himself, or the need for routine lifting or handling obviated: for example, if a heavy patient has to be turned every two hours, the use of a turning bed must be considered. But much remains even after un-

necessary lifting and handling has been rooted out. The question is what effect it has on the body.

It is useful to begin by examining how loads are distributed by the body when starting to lift. The load is gripped and the force at the hands is increased until the load begins to move. At almost the same time, the force at the feet increases: partly as the weight of the load is taken but also from the acceleration of the load. Stand on the bathroom scales to lift and see for yourself. Thus the force of lifting is transmitted through the whole body: from hands to pectoral girdle, along the spine to the pelvis and so to the feet. If you are sitting when you lift, some of the lifting force may be transmitted via the backrest of the seat. If you lift with one hand and support yourself with the free hand, you may be able to offload the spine: as in the Shoulder Lift (see page 79).

Having determined how much of the lifting force is transmitted through the body, the next question concerns the effect on individual parts of the body and the magnitude of the stresses induced: is there a risk of strain and if so how much. This introduces the concept of moments. A moment of force is the tendency of a force to rotate the object to which it is applied. It is measured by multiplying the magnitude of the force by the distance at which it acts from the axis of rotation. Thus the moment of a child sitting at the end of a see-saw equals the moment of the parent who sits nearer the pivot (Fig.1).

Fig 1 *The concept of moments: the see-saw*

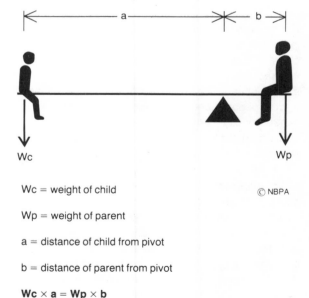

Wc = weight of child   © NBPA

Wp = weight of parent

a = distance of child from pivot

b = distance of parent from pivot

Wc × a = Wp × b

The concept of moments applies to the body. When standing erect, the balls of the feet may act as pivots. If you hold a load at arms' length, the body must lean back to counterbalance the weight of the load held (Fig. 2a). The flexor muscles of the shoulders resist the moment about the shoulder joints. To calculate this moment you need to know the weights of the upper

Fig 2a *Counterbalance*

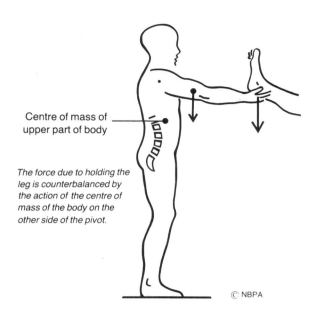

Centre of mass of upper part of body

The force due to holding the leg is counterbalanced by the action of the centre of mass of the body on the other side of the pivot.

© NBPA

Fig 2b *The moment at the shoulder joint*

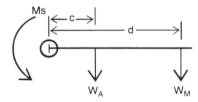

Ms = moment at the shoulder W_A = weight of upper limbs

W_M = weight of load held   d = distance of load from shoulder

c = distance of centre of mass of upper limbs from shoulder

Ms = $W_A \times c + W_M \times d$ © NBPA

The moments of the weight of the upper limbs and load are counterbalanced by the anti-clockwise moment from the shoulder muscles.

limb and of the load; plus the distances of their centres of mass from the shoulder joint. When the resulting force is transmitted down the spine, the lower back muscles resist the moment about the lumbosacral disc: the calculation is shown in **Fig. 2b**. This is precisely what happens when a nurse, for example, is asked to hold a patient's leg up in the plaster room while a splint is being applied.

With all the relevant facts, the weights and their distances from the spinal axis, it then becomes possible to estimate the compressive load on the spine itself (**Fig. 2b, 2c**). The one key factor which is readily understood and felt is that the further a load is from the body, the greater the stress on the back (**Fig. 3**). This should be interpreted in the light of the Manual Handling Operations Regulations 1992 which suggest the guideline figure of 25 kg (55 lb) as the maximum for manual lifting under optimal conditions, close to the body and with the hands between mid-thigh and hip-height.

Fig 2c *Moments about the lower back*

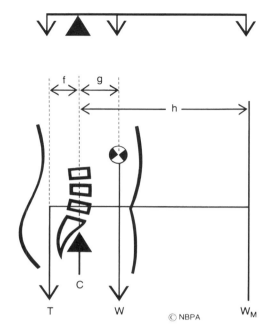

© NBPA

W_M = weight of load (from Fig.2b)   W = weight of upper half of body

T = tension in back muscles

f = horizontal distance between line of section of back muscles and spinal axis

g = horizontal distance between line of action of centre of upper body mass and spinal axis

h = horizontal distance of load from spinal area

$T \times f = W \times g + W_M \times h$

C = the compressive load on the disc $= T + W + W_M$

The loads from the hands and the body's centre of mass give clockwise moments, counteracted by an anti-clockwise moment from the lower back muscles.

Fig 3 *Relationship between load weight and distance from the body*

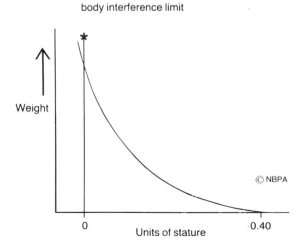

© NBPA

Decrease in the ability to support a weight with increasing distances from the body. Distance from body is given as a proportion of stature.

Body Posture and the Exertion of Force

A lifting action takes the load upwards or vertically: but seldom strictly vertical. This is partly because a lift also requires that the load be moved or carried sideways. The other reason is that a strictly vertical lift is not necessarily easier. Ideally, your feet should be under the load in order to minimise the resulting stress on the back. We teach that the load lifted should be over the area of your stance: the area between your feet (Fig. 4). But we also teach that the

Fig 4 *The area of stance*

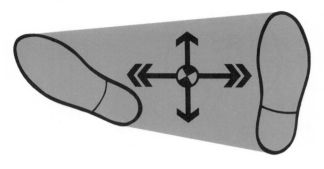

© NBPA

feet should be far enough apart to maintain balance in the direction of movement after the initial lift. Thus the majority of lifts have a horizontal component. And this is consistent with our knowledge of the direction in which the greatest forces can be developed (Grieve & Pheasant 1981).

A vertical lift requires the exertion of muscular strength in order to increase the distance between hands and feet. When the force is directed horizontally, body-weight can be used. Pushing and pulling therefore require muscular control of the posture so that necessary horizontal distance between hands and feet are maintained. But this introduces another factor. You can only push or pull effectively if your feet do not slip. The pushing or pulling force at the hands is matched by the reaction between the feet and the floor. Thus the resistance underfoot may be a limiting factor in any handling or lifting action in which the load is moved sideways.

What is essential is that the lifting posture is in balance. If an attempt is made to lift at the limit of reach, the only way to produce the necessary force may well be to pull at the same time. Then the lifting posture is unstable. The importance of postural stability when lifting can not be too strongly emphasised, especially given the uncertainties of lifting when the load is human (Hollis 1991).

Fatigue and Repetition

We all know that a lot of physical activity makes us tired, and recognise the muscular discomforts associated with heavy work. Doing nothing is also tiring if it involves holding a posture for any length of time. In

fact this kind of 'static work' can cause a feeling of muscular tiredness very much more quickly than active force exertions – 'dynamic work'. It is also true that recovery from static work, so that the same force or posture can be held for the same maximum length of time, also takes much longer than recovery from the exhaustion of dynamic work.

The effect of this fatigue from static work is to reduce the holding time and/or the maximum force you can exert. Frequent short exertions with rest-pauses allow more complete recovery than the same total time of exertion with the same total recovery time. If muscular activity is to continue without pause for an unlimited time, contraction intensity should not exceed about 5% of the maximum.

Fig. 5 illustrates the relation between fatigue and recovery. This example shows how the planning of work may bring about a substantial reduction of the risk of fatigue; plus a more efficient use of working time. So the kinds of jobs where bodily postures and forces have to be maintained should be spread over the work period, to match the demands more closely

Fig 5 *Measurement of dynamic work*

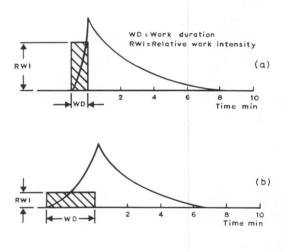

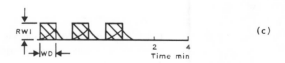

Schematic representation of build-up of fatigue, and recovery in three types of exercise. (a) Very high intensity exercise during 1 min, followed by recovery which in this case took around 9 min. (b) Exercise at 1/3 of previous intensity, performed during 3 min, followed by recovery which took around 7 min. (c) Intermittent exercise consisting of three exercise periods at 1/3 of initial intensity, each performed during 1 min with 1-min pauses interspersed. Note the brief recovery periods.

From Wilson & Corlett 1990. Reproduced with the kind permission of Professor Åsa Kilbom and Taylor & Francis Ltd.

to the body's ability to cope. In just the same way, unnecessary postures should be avoided, e.g. bending when you could sit. If adjustment is available which would give you a better posture, then use it. Also note where the alteration of equipment or the provision of seating or other body support will reduce adverse postures.

For example, if a nurse in the community is stooped over a patient in a low bed for 10 minutes in order to carry out a difficult catheterisation, it will be a few minutes before her back muscles recover their efficiency unless she can quickly mobilise it. Or if two nurses are, unavoidably, required to lift and hold a patient suspended for 3 minutes while his pressure areas are attended to, it could well be 36 minutes before their muscles will be sufficiently recovered to lift another patient safely. When in doubt, it is wise to allow time for recovery using a factor of up to 12 times the duration of exposure.

Repetition is another aspect of body loading which is easily overlooked. When we first start a different job our bodies will adapt to the new regime over the first few days, and this is normal. Note 'the first few days' not the first few months! If there is still discomfort and fatigue which extends into the next week, then there is a good cause for reassessing the workplace and the tasks.

There are many well recognised diseases which can be triggered by repetition, particularly when combined with muscle forces; tenosynovitis of the wrist and 'tennis elbow' are two which are not uncommon. Very frequent loading of the same muscles and tendons, or joints, can create problems by the accumulation of a lot of small loads. As with lifting, the advice is to distribute the loads over time as widely as possible and to note the early onset of discomfort. This last is a warning which should be heeded, and a change of activities instituted to reduce the loading on the affected part.

Individual Factors – Anthropometry

Nurses and carers vary greatly in body height, weight and shape. The variation in height, for example, is illustrated in **Fig. 6**. It shows the range of heights in a population and where the average (the 50th percentile) will lie. Females between 19 and 45 years of age vary from 4'11½" (1515 mm) for the shortest (5th percentile) to 5'7½" (1715 mm) for the tallest (95th percentile) (Pheasant 1986). The variation is about 6% either side of the average.

Variations in body-weight, however, can be as much as 25% either side of the average. In a study of 1,150 females of working age in NW England, the average weight was 134 lb (61 kg) (Troup *et al.* 1987). It varied from 100.5 lb (46 kg) for the 5th percentile to 168 lb (76 kg) for the 95th percentile. Muscle strength can vary even more: maximal isometric lifting strength at

Fig 6 *Histogram of height distribution in the population*

Numbers in
each group

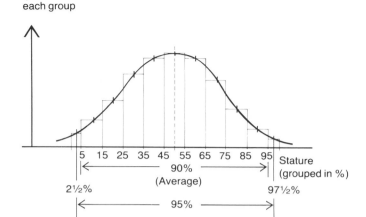

The largest group is average height, because the curve is symmetrical about its mid-point.

© NBPA

waist level in females averaged 55 lb (25 kg) and varied by 45%, from 30 lb (14 kg) for the 5th percentile to 81 lb (37 kg) for the 95th percentile.

Using a dynamic lifting test of the maximum acceptable weight for females to lift, Snook & Ciriello (1991) reported an average of 37 lb (17 kg) for lifting from floor to knuckle height, close to the body, once every minute. For lifting once every eight hours, the average was 62 lb (28 kg). But again the variation was considerable. For the 5th – 95th percentile, variation was 58% for one lift/minute and 56% for one lift every 8 hours. The range of handling strength between the 5th percentile female and the 95th percentile male is shown in **Fig. 7** (Sanchez & Grieve 1992).

This variation in individual body size and strength must be recognised and remembered. The ergonomist must allow for it in any work design. As it is difficult, if not wholly impracticable, to recruit teams of nurses and carers who do not display this large and perfectly normal variation, the workload must be designed to suit at least 90% of the population at risk. For example, it is not practicable to work out duty rotas so that the nurses on duty in a ward at any one time are all within, say, 5 cm of the same height. The workload must be safe for the majority.

The other point which emerges from the difference in the figures for maximal acceptable lift strength (Snook & Ciriello 1991), is that individuals will vary very greatly in what they can comfortably lift; depending on frequency of lift as well as other factors. At the end of the night shift, a nurse may not feel as strong and, in fact, will be found to be relatively weaker than when reporting for duty. The ergonomist must allow for this in the design of work: likewise managers in planning the system of work.

Fig 7a&b *The Measurement and prediction of isometric lifting strength in symmetrical and asymmetrical postures*

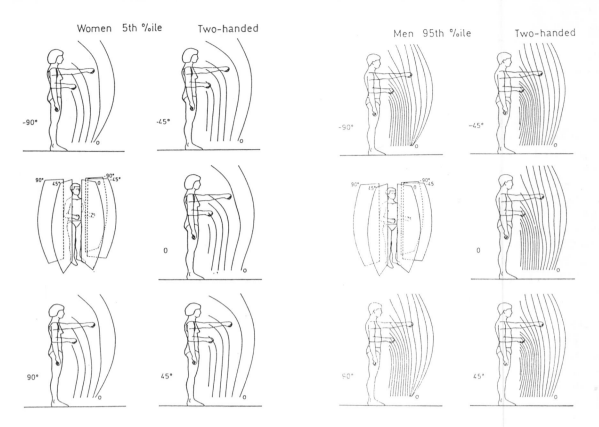

Fig 7a *Lifting isodynes of a person whose body-weight equals that of a 5th percentile female for two-handed exertions. The outermost line represents zero force and each subsequent line an increase of 5 kg.*

Fig 7b *Lifting isodynes of a person whose body-weight equals that of a 95th percentile male for two-handed exertions. The outermost line represents zero force and each subsequent line an increase in 5 kg.*

From Sanchez & Grieve 1992. Reproduced with the kind permission of the authors and Taylor & Francis Ltd.

The Handling Environment

Workspace

Human bodies need room for manoeuvre all around in the course of patient-handling. Nurses and carers have to be keenly aware of the space in which they work. Their handling postures must be stable. They need space behind themselves as well as in the direction they intend to move the patient. They need additional space when using handling equipment. The space must be cleared of obstructions and hazards.

This means taking positive action. All handlers will learn to modify and manipulate the space in which they work; and this is the application of user-ergonomics. The space between chair and commode; the height of the bed; the position of lockers or anything that may get in the way; even the space between beds: the handler must be prepared to optimise. But if the handler has regularly to move beds in order to optimise space, this task itself causes strain. The responsibility then falls on management to find a solution: for instance, reducing the number of beds.

The question of space and access can be critical, particularly in the community. Consider, for instance, a dependent patient sick at home after discharge from hospital: lying in a double bed in a corner of a crowded room. In an emergency there may be no choice for the carer. Before the patient returns from hospital there should be ample time to plan the environment in which the carers will have to work and in which the patient's rehabilitation will have to continue. This is a matter for safe discharge procedure (Department of Health 1989) and the proper communication between the Health Authority Community Nursing Service and the Local Authority Social Services.

For a single bed:

> "The minimum dimension of each bed space should be 2.5 metres by 2.9 metres (long axis of bed) and there should be no intrusion into this space." (Department of Health 1986)

Other Environmental Factors

Visibility is an overriding criterion for safe handling. This imposes a major problem for night staff. The pool of incontinent urine is probably invisible and the staff may have to rely on foresight of the probability, given their knowledge of the patient. But in general, the staff must rely on their powers of observation so that the appearance of anything unusual or unexpected in the handling environment is promptly recognised.

General environmental factors such as noise, temperature and humidity may not directly influence a handling task. But influence it they certainly can, by accelerating the onset of fatigue. In these conditions, rest periods may have to be longer or more frequent.

Clothing

It has been the tradition for women, in hospitals and in the community, to wear skirts. But skirt design follows fashion. In recent decades, skirts have tended to constrain the free movements of the lower limbs: and this has been true even for hospital uniforms some of which are so tight as to prevent both flexion and hip abduction. Many of the handling techniques that are described in the pages that follow require that the nurse or handler can put one knee on the bed and have a foot firmly on the floor at the same time. Although some divided skirts are adequate for handling purposes, trousers have the advantage and are to be recommended not only to the Employing Authorities but to individual nurses and carers.

That the handlers' clothing should have nothing that is likely to catch in the clothing of the patient, should go without saying. The problem may not lie in the clothing itself, or the buttons, badges and belt-buckles, but in what goes into pockets. For it is not so much patient/handler contact that has to be considered but any movement between them when in contact. When the handler is faced with a patient who can no longer be supported on his feet, then the patient must be slid gently to the floor, anything which is likely to catch remains a potential hazard.

The patient's clothing is also a consideration. Many dependent patients need clothing which they can readily manipulate. Those who suffer from urgency of micturition may need clothing that is readily released. Again, it is less easy to obtain a firm hold on a patient who is wearing a nylon nightdress than on one who is wearing a belted skirt or trousers.

Information – Communication

The lack of information relating to patient-handling is a risk factor. In an emergency, there may understandably be too little information. But at no other time. It is obviously a failure of communication if a change in a patient's condition is not reported to the next duty shift. But it is equally a failure of communication if a twenty stone patient is admitted from the waiting list for surgery with postoperative immobilisation with no warning to the ward staff, either of the patient's weight or of the surgeon's precise intentions: in such a case, the problems were clearly foreseeable and

the necessary preparations should have been planned. Such failures of communication are regrettably common but nonetheless inexcusable. Precisely where the communication block arises must be investigated: at some point between medical staff, the admissions office and the ward – all under different administrative staff. A similar tendency for a communications block commonly exists in the community: say between the Local Authority Social Services Department responsible for home care staff and the Health Authority's Community Nursing Service; or between the regular community nurse attending a patient and the nurse who relieves her. Handling problems and their solutions tend not to be shared, and further difficulties may exist over the funding, supply and maintenance of handling equipment: especially hoists.

At another level, communication problems arise from failure of assessment. In patients' Care Plans, for example, there is usually a section under the heading of 'mobility', though seldom one on patient-handling. But it is exceptional for guidelines on how the patient should be handled, supported or moved to receive a mention under any heading whatever in the Care Plan.

Communication between individuals is obviously of basic significance when two or more handlers are engaged in a patient-transfer: see page 53 on the question of timing.

Maintenance

Everything degrades over time: the height-adjustment on beds, the wheels of the commodes or the hoists and their attachments. The need for communication becomes obvious here. The problem is first one of recognition, of routine inspection. But next is the problem of action. For when equipment is out of order, trouble is in the offing. Failure of maintenance is an established factor in the occurrence of accidents. When it occurs, there is an inevitable change of routine; occasionally unheralded. The change of routine creates more work and greater strain and it, too, is a factor in the cause of accidents. It is not uncommon to see a bathroom used to store the wheelchairs that are awaiting repair, causing a major obstacle in the use of the bathroom: a foreseeable source of accident and an increase in the workload.

But many things can be kept running well if they are well maintained. Just as cars are regularly serviced in accordance with the manufacturers' guidelines and in deference to the Department of Transport, the same rule should be applied to everything in hospital or community health services. What matters is partly the efficiency of the routine survey on a planned cycle, but also the chain of communication when a fault is first identified. If a care assistant reports the fault, what plan of action is set in motion and with what effect. A fit subject for the safety audit (see page 42).

Planning of Workload in the Patient's Day

All too often the system of work is reduced to a travesty of crisis management. Nothing is anticipated. Any expedient serves to make do. Two examples show the need for proper organisation and forethought:

- Three nurses were observed dragging an armchair, in which an extremely large patient was seated, for the length of the ward: it was a major struggle. The object was to change the patient's bed position. Why, therefore, was the patient not moved in the bed?

- As part of the night staff's routine, patients in an elderly care ward were toiletted as soon as the staff came on duty. This involved some heavy handling tasks. An observer noted that several of the patients had been toiletted only half an hour previously when the day staff were helping them to bed. In this instance, consideration of the individual's needs would have reduced the nurses' workload.

The Ergonomics Overview

In the preceding part of this chapter, some aspects of ergonomics of direct relevance to health care activities and the handling of patients have been discussed. There are, of course, many other aspects not touched on here which also influence the performance of work. These may be of more or less importance depending on the job being considered.

Readers who wish for a broader knowledge will find useful texts given in the bibliography. For this final section it will be useful if the general ergonomics viewpoint on the investigation and design of work is presented. This will give the reader a framework for further advance, as well as a point of view from which appropriate solutions to problems can be developed.

Ergonomics puts the people doing the job at the centre of the picture, and refers everything to them. It sees efficiency in terms of effective performance which is achieved by being within the capacities of the people concerned. Organisations should have, as their primary purpose, to help those employed to achieve the requirements of the system, and only secondarily for bureaucratic convenience. Managing, to the ergonomist, is creating circumstances whereby people can do their work most effectively, not a system of control over – and monitoring of – people's behaviour.

Obviously people, money, output and quality have to be monitored. However, these are seen in many conventionally organised systems as being achieved by control of use and movement. Ergonomics sees its contribution to the creation of systems whereby the people doing the work – who ultimately create the output and quality – have the best opportunities to monitor and influence these themselves. Management are facilitators, planners and policy makers. The workforce are the creators and achievers, feeding their needs and experiences to the management in a cooperating partnership.

On a smaller scale, when studying a work situation, ergonomists look for mismatches. Where do workloads come from? What causes the fatigue or discomfort? Why are things lifted or pushed? Can people see what they need to see, or reach without bending or stretching up? How many pieces of information do they have to take in, or use to reach a given decision? What is ambiguous or unclear, confusing or conflicting?

Assessment procedures, of which one is given as an example in Chapter 5, are based on these concepts. They use a combination of people's experiences, ergonomics knowledge and measurements to determine a profile of the workplace, around which questions can be asked or dimensions compared.

In one of his Father Brown detective stories, G.K. Chesterton has his characters discussing a lie detector. The discussion has some relevance to our ergonomics way of thinking.

> "Isn't that better evidence than a lot of gabble from witnesses – the evidence of a reliable machine?" said Usher.
> "You always forget", said his companion (Father Brown) "that the reliable machine always has to be worked by an unreliable machine".
> "Why, what do you mean" asked the detective.
> "I mean Man", said Father Brown, "the most unreliable machine I know of."
> (Chesterton 1970)

The ergonomist's job is to set the situation of the machine so that this 'unreliable machine, Man' can use his abilities to ensure that their joint output can be and remains reliable throughout their working lives.

Chapter 4
Epidemiology

Introduction

Patient-handling, or the physical work of lifting, carrying, supporting, moving or otherwise transferring patients and the disabled, remains the commonest source of reported injuries to nurses and carers. Musculoskeletal symptoms, such as backache, remain a major problem. Those who are at risk are the nurses and carers in hospitals and residences where the proportion of dependent people is highest. The last large-scale study in the United Kingdom was published by Stubbs et al. (1983) who estimated that 764,000 days of work were lost by nurses because of back pain. A decade later, there may be fewer nurses at risk. But with the increasing numbers of dependent people in the population and the decline in the number of qualified nurses, the burden falls increasingly on nursing assistants and on carers in the community.

The risk of injury depends on several factors. When assessing this risk, all the contributory factors must be in mind. Table 1 gives the sample of risk factors from the EC Directive. Translated into patient-handling risks, the most significant is the level of physical dependency of the patients and their need for nursing care. Thus geriatric, acute orthopaedic and intensive care wards are the environments in which nurses and carers are at particular risk (Osborne 1978; Sharp 1985; Venning et al. 1987). Similar risks arise in homes for elderly and disabled people. The nurses and carers who do the most patient-handling are again at greater risk and thus the nurses with the higher qualifications are less at risk (Videman et al. 1984; Venning et al. 1987; Jensen 1990). So far as the individual is concerned, the most important risk factor is a previous history of back trouble. Strength and physical fitness is theoretically an important factor though Videman et al. (1989) found this to be of limited importance. But a recent study at Oxford has shown that endurance-strength of the knee-extensor muscles was an indicator (Moffett et al. 1992). Probably of greater importance is a combination of factors. Physical fitness in its general sense is one of them. Another is neuromuscular coordination and motor skills. But a third key factor is the ability to plan the lifting environment. An educational programme was designed in Helsinki to teach student nurses to apply basic ergonomics to the handling environment as well as improve their physical handling skills: the results were promising. The skill with which they could plan and carry out patient-handling tasks could be improved. The follow-up study then demonstrated that those with the greater handling skills were at significantly less risk of injury (Videman et al. 1989).

The risk is greatest in those who are new to the work, learner nurses and recruits to the work of caring. The risk returns, particularly in females with children to look after in addition to the occupational workload, in the early thirties, and this is the time when ill-health retirement, because of persistent back trouble, is at its peak (Videman et al. 1984).

But to determine just how much of the back trouble in nurses and carers is directly caused by the occupation there is a difficulty. Some 15% of the working population, more in females, report that they experience back pain at least once a week (Troup et al. 1987): for the 365 nurses in the study the level was 19%. In a study of 219 nurses, mostly employed in a teaching hospital, Foreman (1988) asked about the presence of back pain at the time of questioning (point prevalence): the highest point prevalence of 92% was for nurses in a geriatric ward and the lowest was 28% in a surgical ward. Though, undoubtedly, back trouble tends to prevail throughout the population, in some occupations the prevalence is higher. In general, back injuries are commoner and backache more prevalent where nurses and health care workers are responsible for high-dependency patients and 'clients'.

The Causes of Back Pain

Backache is as widespread and common a symptom as headache. But occasionally it becomes acutely painful: sometimes because of an accident but often for no apparent reason. The immediate task, medically, is to ensure that the symptoms do not stem from some underlying disease and thus exclude all but the commoner mechanical derangements of the spine. As with all forms of pain, the experience of back pain depends on a disturbance of neurological function and there are four basic causes: primary, secondary, referred and psychosomatic (Wyke 1976).

22 Epidemiology

Table 1 *Reference Factors*

ANNEX I (°)

REFERENCE FACTORS

(Article 3 (2), Article 4 (a) and (b) and Article 6 (2))

1. **Characteristics of the load**

   The manual handling of a load may present a risk particularly of back injury if it is:
   — too heavy or too large,
   — unwieldy or difficult to grasp,
   — unstable or has contents likely to shift,
   — positioned in a manner requiring it to be held or manipulated at a distance from the trunk, or with a bending or twisting of the trunk,
   — likely, because of its contours and/or consistency, to result in injury to workers, particularly in the event of a collision.

2. **Physical effort required**

   A physical effort may present a risk particularly of back injury if it is:
   — too strenuous,
   — only achieved by a twisting movement of the trunk,
   — likely to result in a sudden movement of the load,
   — made with the body in an unstable posture.

3. **Characteristics of the working environment**

   The characteristics of the work environment may increase a risk particularly of back injury if:
   — there is not enough room, in particular vertically, to carry out the activity,
   — the floor is uneven, thus presenting tripping hazards, or is slippery in relation to the worker's footwear,
   — the place of work or the working environment prevents the handling of loads at a safe height or with good posture by the worker,
   — there are variations in the level of the floor or the working surface, requiring the load to be manipulated on different levels,
   — the floor or foot rest is unstable,
   — the temperature, humidity or ventilation is unsuitable.

4. **Requirements of the activity**

   The activity may present a risk particularly of back injury if it entails one or more of the following requirements:
   — over-frequent or over-prolonged physical effort involving in particular the spine,
   - an insufficient bodily rest or recovery period,
   — excessive lifting, lowering or carrying distances,
   — a rate of work imposed by a process which cannot be altered by the worker.

—

Primary Back Pain

Primary back pain arises directly from the tissues of the spine – skin, muscle or muscle fascia, ligaments, periosteum, apophyseal joint capsules, adventitia of blood vessels, dura and dural root sleeves (Fig. 8). These tissues are all supplied with sensory nerves, called nociceptors, whose free nerve endings respond to mechanical and chemical irritation. Primary back pain can therefore be brought about by fatigue and unaccustomed activity, by postural stress, as a

Fig 8 *Structure of the lower spine*

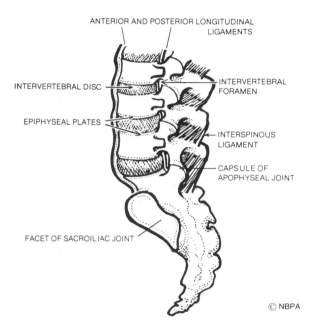

© NBPA

result of trauma and because the tissues are affected by local pathological change such as osteoarthritis. The actual pain is often diffuse and difficult to localise, particularly if its origin is deep. When severe it can become widespread, often being felt in the buttocks and backs of the thighs (McCall *et al.* 1979). But there are two types of tissue in the spine which have no nerve supply and which cannot therefore be

sites for primary back pain: these are the nucleus of the disc together with all but the outermost layers of the annulus fibrosus (Fig. 9) and the cartilage which forms the epiphyseal plates on the surfaces of the vertebral body and which lines the facets of the apophyseal joints. Thus the weight-bearing tissues, the discs and the surfaces of the apophyseal joints may be injured without pain. Often the onset of pain is delayed until the effect of the injury to the disc or facets has secondarily involved neighbouring tissues: delays of twenty-four hours or more after the injury being common.

Fig 9 *Spinal structure – disc*

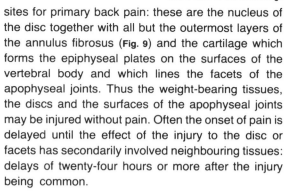

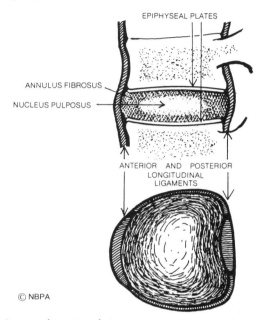

© NBPA

Secondary Back Pain

Secondary back pain arises when the nerves which supply the spine become irritated or when they are stretched or compressed enough to interfere with the blood supply and with the conductivity of their nerve fibres. The nerves at risk are the posterior primary rami of the spinal nerves and the sinuvertebral nerves (Fig. 10) which may be jeopardised by the encroach-

Fig 10 *Vertebra and nerves*

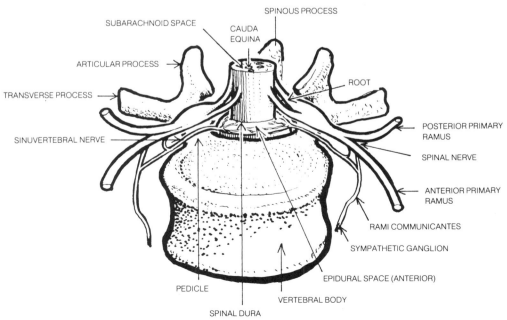

© NBPA

ment of hypertrophic bony growth from the margins of the vertebral body or from the articular processes, or by encroachment from disc degeneration. When these nerves are irritated, the fibres whose conductivity are most at risk are the large, fast-conducting mechanoreceptors (mediating the sensation of touch and movement). Activity in these fibres has an inhibitory effect on nociceptor activity, so providing one of the mechanisms which normally prevent pain from becoming persistent or chronic. Thus when the conductivity of mechanoreceptors is reduced, pain may stay unchecked and this is typical of secondary back pain.

Referred Back Pain

Referred back pain arises not from the tissues of the spine, but from a structure in the abdomen or pelvis, or on the abdominal wall, which is the site of disease. Pain may be referred to that part of the back which has a nerve supply from the same segmental level. Referred pain must be excluded in every case of back symptoms.

Psychosomatic Back Pain

The last in Wyke's classification is psychosomatic back pain: not back pain with so-called functional overlay but back pain arising from psychiatric disturbance, from wanton malingering, and from no other cause. Psychosomatic back pain is thus distinct from the psychological or behavioural changes, such as depression, that are secondary to the back pain itself. It is rare.

Pain in the Leg

Pain in the leg is commonly associated with back pain as in 36 per cent of the nurses in the sample reported by Lloyd and Breen (1985). In many cases of severe primary back pain, the associated leg pain is referred from the back (McCall *et al.* 1979): this probably

represents the majority of cases but without accurate diagnosis the proportion remains uncertain.

A number of those with pain in the leg have a condition equivalent to secondary back pain. In other words, there is a source of irritation in the lower back affecting the nerve supply of the lower limb: those parts of the nerve roots which go to form the anterior primary ramus of the spinal nerve. Commonly the roots affected are the L4, L5 and S1 which join the sacral plexus and form the sciatic nerve (**Fig. 11**).

Fig 11 *Sciatic nerve*

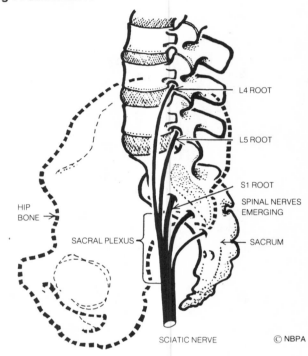

In many forms of root involvement, this is just an irritative lesion affecting the root, causing pain in the distribution of the sciatic nerve and restricting those movements which stretch the nerve. Where this is an intervertebral disc prolapse, for example, which stretches and angulates the root from its normal path (**Fig. 12**), the signs of root tension may be sup-

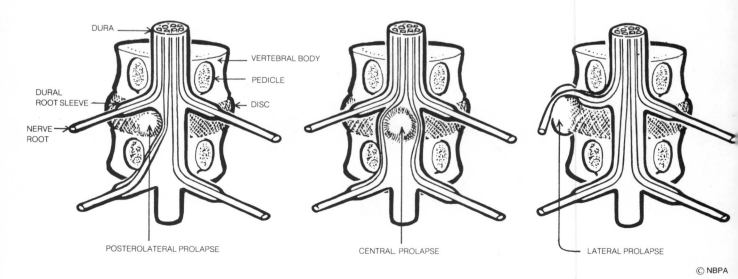

Fig 12 *Intervertebral disc prolapses showing how the root is stretched and augulated from its normal path by the prolapsed material*

plemented by signs of diminished sensation, muscle power or reflex response in the lower limbs. In other cases the root may become compressed particularly on extending or on flexing to the affected side and then symptoms of numbness and weakness may be more severe. The likelihood of nerve root involvement in any given case of back pain is partly a function of the size and shape of the spinal canal and intervertebral foramina; and thus depends on the space available for the nerve roots in the presence of an existing disc prolapse or of an existing amount of hypertropic, degenerative encroachment. Those with narrow or stenotic spines are more liable to sciatic symptoms in the presence of any given lumbar spinal disorder (Porter *et al.* 1980).

Chronic Back Pain

Back pain has a multifactorial aetiology. Not only is there a host of possible contributory factors: these factors tend to interact. Failure to recover spontaneously from an acute episode is therefore very common. Sometimes this is because the underlying reason for the initial episode of pain has not been discovered. Another reason is that treatment has relied on prolonged periods of rest rather than on prompt and active rehabilitation. The chronic back pain patient comes to rely on painkillers and slowly becomes more unfit and thus more susceptible to further trouble.

Of great importance clinically is the psychological effect of the back pain itself. The experience of acute back pain may provoke fear: fear of recurrence, fear that there is some underlying disease, fear that it may not recover. Secondarily, this may cause depression. Thus the pain may acquire a psychogenic component and there is a risk, in some patients, that the experience of back pain may lead to exaggerated pain perception and illness behaviour (Waddell *et al.* 1984): often the case when the perfectly natural initial fear engendered by the pain goes unrecognised and untreated (Troup & Videman 1989). Even then, recovery from prolonged back pain may still be hindered by factors that tend to reinforce the pain: litigation and compensation claims being amongst the better known (Greenough & Fraser 1989).

Back Pain At Work

From the section above on the causes of back pain, it is an inescapable fact that back pain can seldom be attributed to a single cause. In the majority of cases of acute back pain, the onset is not attributed to any kind of injury (Lloyd & Troup 1983), though occupational factors often serve as triggers to provoke an attack. Sometimes, the association between the onset of pain and the task at which the individual was engaged at the time is a matter of coincidence. Nonetheless, there is a variety of physical factors at work that are recognised as contributory or causal factors.

Unaccustomed Work

Unaccustomed work entailing bending or spells of work which are heavier than usual are common, and normal causes of back pain (Magora 1970a, 1970b, 1972, 1973; Biering-Sørensen 1983). It requires time to adapt to new work, particularly if new psychomotor skills have to be learnt, as when first handling patients. This is analogous to the epidemic of sports injuries at the beginning of every season (Williams and McKibbin 1978). Moreover, spells of exceptionally heavy work may predispose people to back injury (Anderson and Sweetman 1980). One of the major reasons for exposure to unaccustomed work is the change of routine: due to unexpected staff shortages, disruption of ward practices or mechanical failure of equipment. Whenever such changes in workload occur, the attendant risks should be recognised.

Postural Stress

Postural stress is an equally common cause of back pain (Riihimäki 1990). Much of the prevalence of back pain, particularly in high-dependency wards and residences, can be ascribed to postural stress. Nurses and carers spend long periods stooped over the job. This is especially so when attending to patients in bed; it applies also to caring for those who are wheelchair-bound and for children. The immediate consequence of postural stress is muscular fatigue. It requires a level of isometric tension that, particularly in muscles enclosed within a potentially tight fascial sheath, may cause ischæmia. It is believed that this can happen in the muscles of the back and their contractility reduced. They need time to recover. The second consequence is the resulting static load on the spine and its duration: the outcome, as with repeated lifting, is discal narrowing and shrinkage of stature (Corlett 1990). Postural stress and prolonged muscle tension also contribute to the more general levels of stress, fatigue or tiredness to which nurses and carers may be exposed. Backache is to be expected. Typically, the nurse spends periods leaning over the patient's bed: recording blood pressures, giving intravenous drugs or carrying out dressings on the underside of patient's legs. It is postural stress that is the likely origin of the syndrome known as 'Nurses' Back' (Figs 13, 14, 15, 16).

The Risks of the Twisted Back

There is one further point to consider. The intervertebral disc consists of a nucleus pulposus which is enclosed in the annulus fibrosus, a ligament of great strength in which alternate layers of fibres are arranged more or less at right angles to each other and at an oblique angle to the vertebral bodies (Fig.17). This gives the normal disc great strength; it is usually the vertebral body which fails first in severe injury (Roaf 1960). When the disc is compressed it tends to bulge as intradiscal pressure rises and the tension in the annulus fibrosus increases. If under a given compressive load, the spine is then rotated or laterally flexed the tension in the annulus is accentu-

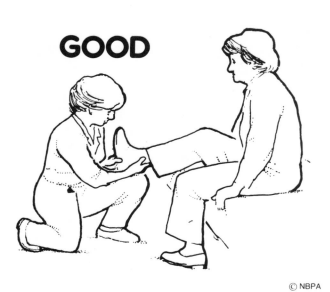

GOOD

© NBPA

Fig 13 *Example of GOOD and BAD posture*

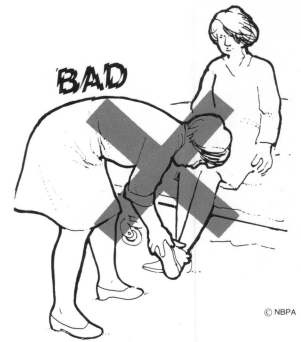

BAD

© NBPA

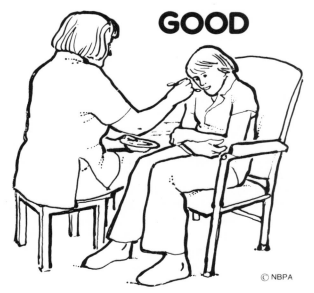

GOOD

© NBPA

Fig 14 *Example of GOOD and BAD posture*

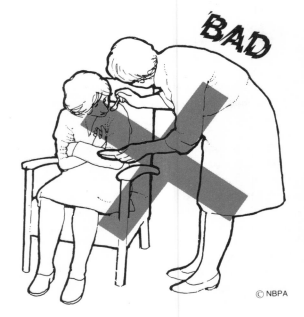

BAD

© NBPA

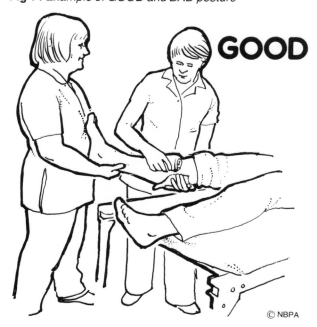

GOOD

© NBPA

Fig 15 *Example of GOOD and BAD posture*

BAD

© NBPA

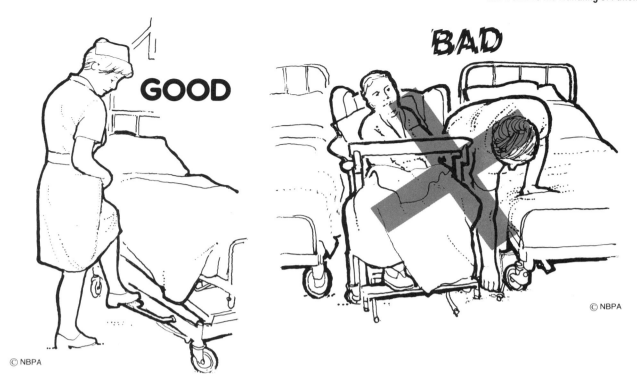

Fig 16 *Example of GOOD and BAD posture*

ated and intradiscal pressure is further increased. This is a major risk if the disc is degenerating and rotation-injuries themselves are causes of degeneration (Farfan 1977).

Back Injuries

To appreciate the causes of back injuries, it is essential to understand the mechanism. The first question concerns what work the casualty was doing at the material time e.g. moving a walking patient. The second question is about the movements and activities at the moment when something went wrong e.g. walking on the patient's left side, holding his left wrist with her left hand and with her right hand round the patient's back. Then comes the key question: what was **the first unforeseen event?**, i.e. what went wrong? Then the sequence of events that follow can be set out and the mechanism of injury determined.

The Vulnerable Back

But with many back injuries, the first unforeseen event was the back pain itself. Nothing had gone wrong up to the moment at which the pain started. Often, the casualty on these occasions has a vulnerable back, but the question is why. Vulnerable because unaccustomed to the work or unfit; vulnerable because of the preceding workload; or vulnerable because of an underlying weakness and the resistance to injury reduced by, for example, advanced degenerative changes.

The preceding workload may, in some circumstances, reduce the resistance of a healthy back to

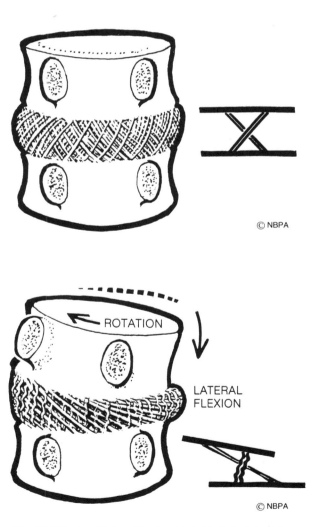

Fig 17 *Effects of lateral flexion and rotation showing increased tension distributed in part of the annulus fibrosus.*

injury. Exposure to repeated minor traumata from unsafe lifting practices over a long period is one example. On the shorter term, mechanical tissue-fatigue may be induced by the immediately preceding workload, thus decreasing the resistance to injury (Hirsch 1955; Brinckmann *et al.* 1988). Here, the phenomenon of the 'creep-effect' must be considered (Kazarian 1975; Köller *et al.* 1981) in which the disc gradually narrows, stiffens and becomes more susceptible to injury. It can be induced by the frequency of heavy lifting, by exposure to postural stress, with no rest-pauses or time for recovery; or by a combination of these factors. At one time, the phenomenon of the 'creep-effect' could only be studied under experimental conditions but now it can be assessed indirectly by measurements of stature (Corlett *et al.* 1987) and a pilot study has been made of nursing activities (Foreman 1988; Foreman *et al.* 1988).

External Factors

But occupationally induced back pain may not necessarily stem from the physical workload, the working posture or any calculable risk of injury. Other factors may also contribute. Monotony, stress at work and want of job-satisfaction have been identified by Magnusson *et al.* (1990) to lead to 'fatigue injuries'; while another study has identified the want of enjoyment of work as a factor that may increase the risk of injury by as much as two and a half times (Bigos *et al.* 1991).

Chapter 5
Assessing the Handling Risk

Introduction

Assessment of risk depends on knowledge or fore-sight of what is or may be unsafe. The requirement to make the assessment affects all nursing and care staff. The overall responsibility for the safety of the individuals at risk by reason of their occupation rests largely with management at every level. The specific responsibility for each handling task lies with the individual nurse or carer. It is she who has to decide the safe and appropriate way to carry out the task and call for such assistance or equipment as may be necessary. Managers who are at a remove from the immediate practicalities of risk assessment have a duty to respond to the problems revealed by assessments. They also have a duty to investigate the accidents and injuries that occur.

By 1992, it will be a statutory requirement to assess the risk of lifting, supporting, carrying patients or disabled persons when assisting them in their movements and transfers. Table 1 on page 22 gives the framework for assessment. But the characteristics of the load in patient-handling are more complex.

- Most patients are too heavy or too large to be lifted bodily.

- All patients, compared with the industrial load, are unwieldy and difficult to grasp.

- Most dependent patients are potentially unstable and some are liable to unexpected movements.

- Patients have frequently to be moved closer before any lift or transfer is possible.

- And though collisions when patient-handling do occur, most of the risk to 'workers' arises, not from the shape or contours of the load but from the physical behaviour of the patient.

The weight and size of patients who have, inescapably, to be lifted and who can not assist in the movement or transfer, requires that lifting equipment be used. In the event that the equipment is unobtainable or impracticable, the usual expedient is to recruit a sufficient number of handlers to share the load. This is a reasonable aim if the load were to be shared equally. Take, for example, a patient who is 5′ 4″ tall (160 cm) and weighs 210 lb (95.5 kg). Most of the weight is in the middle. But there is not room between handlers to share it. The handlers at head and feet invariably have the easier shares. A taller, 15 stone patient may be easier. But there is no way in which a truly obese patient can be lifted manually with reasonable safety. If for no other reason, the larger the patient's girth, the greater the difficulty in getting any grip.

The factors to be considered in assessing the risks in patient-handling are set down in the checklist in Table 2.

Investigating Patient-handling Injuries

In an established work setting, the risk of injury can be assessed also from the occurrence of previous injuries and accidents arising from patient-handling. At present, the statutory duty to report accidents does not extend beyond the need to report. The preventive value of the reporting system is presumed, generally without justification. Yet the need for investigations into the cause of injuries associated with patient-handling has been identified in recommendations in both previous editions of this Guide and in *The Lifting of Patients in the Health Services* from the Health Services Advisory Committee, published by HMSO in 1984. Thus an employer may be held to be negligent when reports of previous injuries are judged to have been ignored, so failing to take steps to avoid later injuries. The Reporting of Injuries, Diseases and Dangerous Occurrences Regulations (RIDDOR) to the Health and Safety Executive is the official source of accident data. But it is not a comprehensive source; nor can the data be taken as representative. On page 42 in the 1988/1989 Annual Report of the Health and Safety Commission it is stated that:

"Inspectors noted a continuing failure by some health authorities to report all relevant accidents as required by RIDDOR. Notices have

Table 2

Checklist for Assessment in Patient-Handling

1. Purpose:
    > the starting and ending points in the lift or transfer
    > task frequency
    > task duration

2. The Patient Data:
    > diagnosis
    > weight, height and shape;
    > ability to assist and liability to fatigue or pain;
    > physical constraints (tubes, splints, traction etc.)
    > behavioural constraints
    > clothing

3. Environmental:
    > furniture: its adjustment and condition
    > handling equipment: access, appropriate attachments
    > space: potential obstructions
    > handler's clothing
    > underfoot stability

4. Selection of Lifting or Transfer Technique:
    > mechanical; assisted manual; or manual.
    >> if manual, number of staff required
    > lifting/handling requirement
    >> vertical lifting
    >> horizontal transfer
    >> support phase
    >> additional tasks while handling (insertion of bedpan, dress adjustment, cleaning etc.)
    > lifting/handling posture
    >> symmetrical
    >> straight back (i.e. not twisted or rotated)
    >> stance

5. Equipment Required:
    > fixed hoist and its attachments
    > mobile hoist, its adjustments and attachments
    > seat-lift
    > handling or transfer equipment
    >> for use by patient
    >> for handlers

6. The Handlers:
    > fitness for the task
    > freshness or fatigue
    > experience with the patient
    > experience with the handling team
    > handling skill
    > familiarity with lifting/handling equipment

7. Action:
    > entry in the Care Plan
    > reassessment *pro re nata*

© NBPA

been served requiring reporting procedures to be set up and two authorities were prosecuted following failure to respond to advice."

So far as injuries and accidents associated with patient-handling are concerned, the question is whether the standard reporting procedures are adequate. It is by no means universal for accident report forms to include a section to state what action was taken. It is a matter of chance if the name of the patient or 'client' involved in the injury is recorded. It is exceptional for the actual patient-handling technique to be identified. One of the difficulties in the past has been the want of an accident-model, in which the accident process can be viewed.

MAIM, the Merseyside Accident Information Model (Troup et al. 1988), which relies on identification of the first unforeseen event perceived by the casualty, has been adapted to the investigation of patient-handling injuries. The following categories of data are required:

- name, age, occupation of the casualty;
- date, time and location of the injury;
- name, diagnosis, mental condition, physical dependency and weight of the patient;
- activity or procedure at the time of injury;
- identity of other handlers;
- mechanical equipment and furniture in use;
- the first unforeseen event;
- the movement at 'the first unforeseen event' and the handling technique in use at the material time;
- the nature of the injury.

These data can readily be supplemented by reference to the Care Plan and the nursing record for the patient. Prospectively, they can be supplemented by a follow-up of the injured person and by a record of the preventive action taken.

Once these basic facts have been recorded, the key question is 'what went wrong in the sequence of events leading to the injury?'. The need is to identify the first unforeseen event as perceived by the injured person (Manning et al. 1984; Troup et al. 1988). Often, the first unforeseen event was the occurrence of pain: thus no true accident but a question of overload or vulnerability may still remain. Alternatively, something happened before the occurrence of pain and this has to be identified because it served as the 'trigger' for what followed. If the triggering event was foreseeable and not an accident 'out of the blue', then it could have been prevented.

The accident investigator must begin by setting the scene with date, time and location and by identifying the individuals involved; the handlers, the patient and witnesses; and the activity in which they were engaged. But then the essential question of the first unforeseen event must now be answered and further questions arise from this first event. What was the movement of the handler at or immediately before that first event. Thus if the first event perceived by the handler was that the patient's knees gave way, the sequence can then be followed logically to the injury itself: caused, say, by the patient landing on top of the handler after they had both fallen to the floor. At each stage, at each event, there is an implicit question of whether the accident process might have been halted and the injury prevented. Ideally, steps might have been taken to ensure that the patient's knees did not give way – so how was the patient being supported? Or having started to give way, might the knees not have been blocked? If the patient could not safely be held upright, might he not have been let fall gently to the floor under proper control?

If, for example, the accident location for the falling patient was a bathroom in which there was little room for manoeuvre and in which it was imperative to stop the patient from falling, prevention falls within the ergonomic sphere: either in terms of redesigning the bathroom or recasting the Care Plan for the patient.

To take a second example of a nurse who feels unexpected pain during a manoeuvre in which nothing had otherwise gone wrong, the questions concern the probability of overload and the possibility of the injured nurse being vulnerable; either because of mechanical and physiological fatigue or from an underlying weakness. Here a combination of preventive approaches may be called for.

Thus as a working hypothesis, the accident investigator must consider whether the events might each have been foreseen and so circumvented. Although the variety of contributory factors may seem complex, the analysis based on identification of the first unforeseen event is simple and logical. The prevention of injuries while patient-handling thus depends on reliable and practical information. But the investigation must be prompt, while the facts are fresh and while the documents such as the Care Plan are still available.

It may take longer to understand the mechanism of injury and the contributory factors using this in-depth approach to accident investigation than when filling in the traditional accident report form, but its potential benefits are infinitely greater. Moreover, practical experience of this system of investigation suggests that the nub of the problem can be revealed within 5-10 minutes in each case.

WARNING

Unsafe Lifting Practices

It is unsafe to lift at arms' length, at a distance from the body, either in front of or to one side of the knees: because you are at a mechanical disadvantage when applying manual forces and because you are at the limit of postural stability. You are at risk of overstrain or overload and you can readily lose balance.

But, regrettably, there are a number of unsafe patient-handling methods that are still in routine use. **They have long been condemned and should be proscribed.** All nurses and carers should be enjoined to beware of them. Just three examples are given and for each of them, there is a wide variety of safe and more comfortable alternatives.

The following three lifts are mentioned here only to condemn them.

The Orthodox Lift

This was the traditional method whereby two nurses stood either side of the bed to lift a patient on the clasped wrists of the nurses under the patients back and thighs (Fig. 18). It would be an unstable lift save for the bed on which the nurses must lean to prevent them falling forward. Their forearms have to be inserted under the patient and they must lift at arms' length: thus inducing a major flexion/compression strain on the lumbar spine. They must then lift sideways: adding a lateral torque to the flexion/compression of the lumbar vertebrae. It transgresses all the rules of safe lifting.

The Drag Lift

The Drag Lift ((Fig. 19) refers to the method of lifting or supporting a patient by his armpits on the crooks of the nurses' elbows. It is performed by two handlers, one on each side of the patient: sometimes to lift a patient up the bed, sometimes to lift a patient from his chair or even from the floor, and then to support the patient while manoeuvring him from A to B. To lift a patient by the armpits is, at best, uncomfortable. For a patient with frail or painful shoulders it is cruel. For a patient who is arthritic or weakened by a stroke, there is a risk of injury to the patient (Hollis 1991).

Moreover, the use of the Drag Lift prevents the patient from using his arms to assist.

The handler is also at risk. To lift a patient by his armpit on the handler's elbow requires her to lift asymmetrically on one side of her body: almost invariably to one side of her knees. It is therefore a potentially unstable lift. It is virtually impossible to keep the back straight. Should anything go wrong, for instance when the patient unexpectedly offers resistance, there is an immediate risk of injury and loss of balance. When two handlers support a patient with the Drag Lift while manoeuvring and turning (Fig. 20 a-c), they are in no position to control the patient in the event of something going wrong: the patient sitting down prematurely or collapsing. Before they can block the patient's knees and control his posture, they must first adjust both their stance and their grip of the patient – not always easy if the patient then clamps the handler's arm against his chest.

Thus the Drag Lift is unsafe on several counts. It is potentially harmful for the patient and biomechanically unsound for the handler. In addition, the discomfort for patients often provokes them to retaliate: not only clasping and gripping the handlers' arms and resisting, but sometimes throwing themselves back, sitting down unexpectedly or even deliberately lifting their feet from the ground.

Lifting with the Patient's Arms round the Handler's Neck

When a handler chooses to lift a patient from the back of a chair with her arms under the patient's shoulders and her hands round the back, she is at risk, especially if lifting from the back of a low chair. The risk is much greater if the patient is permitted or encouraged to put his arms round her neck. First, she is lifting at arms' length well in front of the area of her stance; and, of course, her back is bent forward. The only way she can get the patient to his feet is by throwing herself backwards. She has no control over the patient's lower back or pelvis. If something goes wrong in the course of the lift, and the patient pulls, or puts any weight, on the handler's neck: injury is foreseeable. If it is expedient to let a patient hold the handler in any way, it should be by the handler's belt: but only if there is nothing else such as the armrests of the chair for the patient to push on.

Fig 20a-c *Drag lift from chair*

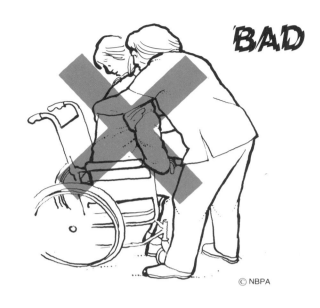

(a)

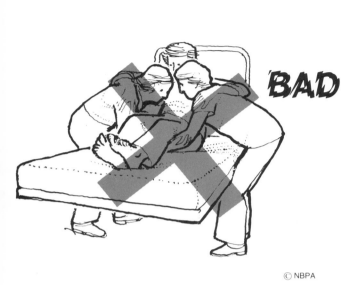

Fig 18 *Orthodox lift*

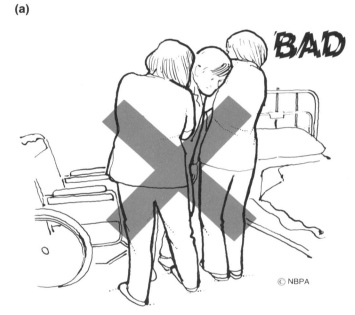

(b)

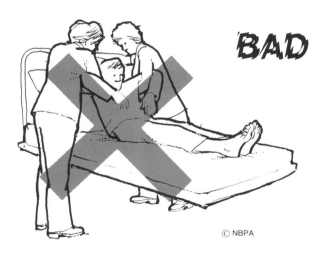

Fig 19 *Drag lift*

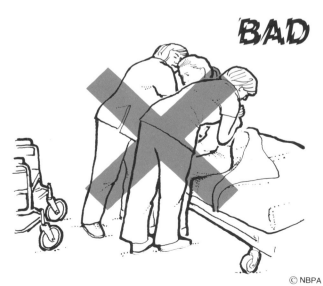

(c)

Chapter 6
Preventative
Approaches

Introduction

Ergonomics, safety-training, pre-employment health screening, treatment at work and the implementation of official guidelines may be considered in isolation, but only in order to understand and define them. They are, or should be, inseparable and it is **ergonomics** that binds them together.

Ergonomics

The subject of ergonomics is dealt with more fully in Chapter 3. The significance of ergonomics to the prevention of injuries and accidents associated with patient-handling is that when a system of work is ergonomically satisfactory, it should be safe. Ergonomic intervention in an existing workplace should lead first to a more efficient system of work and also to a safer one. As with most safety interventions, there should be a cost-benefit.

Safety-training and Housekeeping

Safety-training has two components. The first has a general application and is based on the principles of good housekeeping: ensuring that the environment for patient-handling is clean and uncluttered, that the equipment is in proper working order, that the means of communication are kept open. This aspect of training relies on the development of a keen sense of safety awareness. It is essential that defects and shortcomings are promptly recognised and reported. It is, however, mandatory that such safety-training is backed by a system of response from management. Safety standards can only be maintained if the feedback on safety is met with prompt action (Saari 1987).

The second component of safety-training deals specifically with the practical aspects of patient-handling: partly a question of instruction on how to select the best technique for the specific purpose and how to prepare the handling environment; and partly a matter of practical instruction in the handling skills. But it must be appreciated that no amount of practical skill will protect a handler from an unsafe or ill-designed handling environment. An understanding of basic ergonomics is therefore an essential feature of all safety-training.

Pre-employment Health Screening

Pre-employment health screening is a standard procedure and the question is what proportion of recruits can reasonably be accepted for work requiring patient-handling. When the patient-handling environment is safe and ergonomically satisfactory, the need for major physical exertion on the part of the handler should be largely removed. Thus the majority of recruits to nursing and caring should be physically capable: certainly when the lifting and handling requirements are predictable. But patients do not invariably behave predictably and their condition may fluctuate. So, though the recruit may not require more than average strength, a reasonable standard of physical health and adaptability is essential.

There are, as yet, few reliable tests which have predictive value for back pain or back injury other than the history of previous back trouble (Troup et al. 1987; Videman et al. 1989). In someone who has never experienced back pain there is little to go on. But Biering-Sørensen (1984) has reported the value of an endurance test of the back extensor muscles and Moffett et al. (1992) have identified a similar test of the knee-extensors. These studies may offer some pointers for the future. The value of such tests may reside in more general interpretations of physical fitness. Given the evidence that patient-handling skills are themselves a protection from injury (Videman et al. 1989), what may be needed in pre-employment screening for nurses and carers are tests of neuromuscular coordination and body awareness.

At present, given the dearth of tests of proven reliability and given the shortage of nursing and caring staff, it is reasonable – indeed essential – to accept recruits but to supervise them closely for their capacity to acquire patient-handling skills and their capacity to adapt physiologically to the work. A broad perspective is unavoidable, given the proportion of the population who may be called upon to care for others. It is therefore not enough to confine the pre-employment screening to a simple battery of questions and tests at or before starting the job. After initial screening it is only possible to say that an individual is fit for work, subject to a successful response to training and to a physiological adaptation to the work. Occupational Health Staff therefore have a duty to reassess during the first few months. In-service supervision and assessment of skills during this period are mandatory; and any problems that arise have to be investigated. For it is during this period of adaptation during the first few weeks of employment that the risks are greatest.

Treatment at Work

The preventive value of offering treatment at work for those engaged in patient-handling depends on the prompt identification of need. Work-related symptoms and injuries deserve immediate investigation. Moreover, the cost-benefits of providing treatment at work arise from reduction of the need for sickness absence (Versloot *et al.* 1992); the reduction of potentially harmful effects of rest and inactivity (Deyo *et al.* 1986); and the opportunity for prompt investigation of the cause of incapacity. And today the physiotherapist in Occupational Health relies increasingly on ergonomic intervention as a therapeutic tool.

Back Schools

Many of the larger organisations have established special clinics for the rehabilitation of people with back trouble and they have been successful. But their role may well be extended to provide a service for the symptom free. It is widely believed, for example, that nurses and carers should act positively to keep themselves fit for their work; that there is a risk of injury particularly in those who arrive at work with their muscles still stiff from sleep or who may have to tackle patient-handling tasks after a spell of sedentary work. Although there is no evidence of its value in preventing injuries, it is theoretically sound. The problem is partly one of organisation, but also one of acceptance by those who are supposedly at risk.

Chapter 7
The Management Responsibility:

Implementation of a Patient-handling Policy by the Employing Authority

Assessment of a Patient-handling Need and the Development of Care Plans

The introduction of the problem oriented approach into nursing practice (Nursing, Midwives and Health Visitors Rules Approval Order 1983) requires that patient's problems are assessed on admission and a plan of care developed. An important part of this assessment should include the patient's handling needs and this is now a legal requirement. While it is primarily a nursing responsibility, to be carried out by a Registered Nurse who will have ongoing care of the patient, or by a nursing student working under her supervision, it may be helpful to enlist other professional staff, particularly physiotherapists to contribute to this assessment, as well as a spouse or relative who has been supporting the patient at home. Where it is evident that the handling problems are going to be of some magnitude, a team of experienced personnel should make an assessment and plan of care as soon as possible after admission, but the admitting nurse is still accountable for making an initial assessment and obtaining any necessary equipment.

The nurse making the first assessment of a newly referred patient in the community has similar responsibilities and will enlist the help of other disciplines where appropriate. It is likewise for officers in charge of residential homes to make a note of new residents' mobility problems and give written guidance to their staff on how to help them. While the format of the assessment will depend on the nursing model being used, it should include the following aspects:

- weight
- main disability and specific difficulties in moving
- capabilities
- sensory loss
- state of feet
- specific pain or fear
- understanding
- coping systems prior to admission, i.e. help from relative, self-help systems, equipment in use, etc.

Scoring systems for mobility, independence in daily living, and risk of pressure sores may be useful.

See Fig. 21 for an example of a form which may be adapted as necessary and used for a patient-handling assessment:

- 'Patient's comprehension' should include such items as inability to carry out instructions, deafness, disorientation, cannot speak but understands etc.

- 'Behaviour which may affect' should include such items as loss of confidence, unpredictability, tendency to hit out, poor/good motivation, prone to sudden loss of balance etc.

- A rating such as Green's Patient Handling Scale (Green & McCay 1989) or the Hayne Movement Hazard Code (MHC) can be inserted if in local use (Hayne 1986).

Fig 21 *Example of patient-handling assessment form*

Handling Assessment for Patients who are not Independent

Patient Details (insert label)

```
                    12345X
    Mrs. Smith
    31 Park Road
    Teddington
    TW11 OAB
```

Disability/weakness/deformity

Rheumatoid Arthritis for 20 years

Handling constraints

Pain	*knees very painful*
Skin lesions	*Papery Skin*
Infusions etc.	
Other	
Rating	*2 * B (MHC)*

Problems and capabilities

Walking	*Gets about home with husbands support*
Standing	*can stand from high chair with help*
Toiletting	*needs a raised toilet seat*
Transfers to/from bed	*holds husband round waist and shuffles round*
Movement in bed	*can wriggle up bed but cannot turn over*

Weight: *8st 12lb*

Body Shape:

Tall ☐	Medium height ☑	Obese ☐
Short ☐	Average weight ☐	Thin ☑

Patient's comprehension

No problems

Behaviour which may affect

knows her own limitations + has own routine for coping

History of falls?   Y ☐ N ☑

Equipment normally used by patient

Walking frame
Walking belt
Raised toilet seat

Signature: *L Brown*

Grade: *Rgn*

Date: *2·6·92*

How to use this form

It should be completed within twenty-four hours of patient admission/operation and kept with the nursing assessment sheet.

Main problems together with handling strategy and equipment to be used should be entered into the patient's Care Plan and evaluated on a regular basis.

© NBPA

When the assessment has been made, taking into consideration all the relevant activities of living and self care objectives the problem should be described in very specific terms on the patient's Care Plan, and short and long-term goals negotiated with the patient where appropriate.

In Table 3, for example are the short and long-term goals and nursing instructions for an elderly arthritic lady who has come in for surgery:

This sort of Care Plan will eliminate the unnecessary lifting and handling by the nursing staff which so often destroys a patient's independence, thus putting more burden on the staff or husband in the long-term; it will also hasten his rehabilitation by keeping goals in sight.

The nursing instructions should identify:

- The number of nurses required when handling a patient.

- The method and/or equipment to be used.

- What the patient is expected to do.

- Specific reminders such as 'important to block knees' or 'do not exert pressure on painful left shoulder' are helpful.

Particular hazards must also be identified: e.g. the patient who is prone to fall, and advice given as to his management. Fluctuations in patient performance or variation in nursing skills may require that instructions are written as guidance rather than orders; they should then address the needs of the least skilled and experienced members of staff. But where there is a major handling hazard, the instructions should be absolutely definite: e.g. 'Mr M must not be moved unless four nurses are present' or 'Mr M must only be lifted out of bed with a hoist'.

The Care Plan must be available to all staff who will be handling the patient, and kept near to him, for quick reference. It is essential that patient progress is evaluated regularly by the team and the Plan kept up to date. An out of date Care Plan is highly dangerous and could result in injury to an inexperienced member of staff.

Daily Record

Realistic evaluation will depend on the accuracy of the daily record, which should make reference to:

- patient performance.

- difficulties encountered.

- input from physiotherapist, occupational therapist or relative.

Comments from night staff are especially useful, as patient performance is often quite different at night. An instruction for the day staff may not be feasible at night; the night team should be expected to incorporate night problems and appropriate instructions into the Care Plan.

Preparation for Discharge

Preparation for discharge should follow the recommendation of Department of Health Circular HC(89)5.

Where a handling problem has been identified for a patient in hospital, the handling needs of that patient must be addressed in the discharge plan and provision made well in advance of the discharge date for any equipment, home adaptations or patient/relative teaching required. For example, if a patient is learning to use a sliding board to transfer from bed to chair, he should not be discharged until he has mastered this skill and his carer has been shown how to assist if necessary; or, if a hoist will be required, discharge must be delayed until the right model of hoist and sling has been installed; compatibility with the patient's furniture confirmed and carers shown how to use it.

Occupational therapists, physiotherapists and social workers may all be involved in the discharge planning, but it is essential that one person co-ordinates the arrangements and checks that they have been completed before discharge. It may be appropriate to invite the community nurse to a pre-discharge conference. Similarly, information from the primary care team and relatives should be sought and incorporated into the hospital Care Plan where there has been a long standing mobility problem before admission.

Ward/Primary Care Team Management Issues

Quality standards for patient-handling should be written at a local level as well as for the employing authority.

Important issues to be addressed in these standards are:

- adequate support and supervision for students when handling patients, taking into account the individual's level of experience and skill;

- provision of learning and 'reminder' material, such as books and posters;

- availability of appropriate equipment and firm leadership in bringing it into use;

- a methodical recording system to ensure that every member of the team has been shown by a competent operator how to use the equipment;

- support and encouragement of local patient-handling trainers;

- planning of the patients's day so that handling tasks are reduced to a minimum;

Table 3 *Excerpt from a patient Care Plan*

Problem	Desired Outcome	Nursing Instructions
2/6/92 Mrs S. has severe pain in her knees but manages to walk about the house with a walking frame and husband's support. 4/6/92 Has had difficulty in getting to her feet since operation	That Mrs S's level of mobility should be maintained while in hospital. She aims to stand-up from chair independently and walk out to toilet with one nurse supporting by Day 10. **Review Daily**	~~2/6/92~~ chair or as far as she feels able, using walking frame and wearing belt with one nurse supporting. ~~4/6/92~~ leans forward and pushes up on bed or chair to stand. 9/6/92 Now walking out to toilet with frame and one nurse escorting.

- organisation of the workload so that no one member of staff has an excessive patient-handling load, leading to cumulative strain;

- organisation of duty rotas so that no individual member of staff works excessively long hours or an excessive number of consecutive days, in order to reduce the likelihood of cumulative strain occurring;

- prompt action following reports of handling hazards or dangers in the working environment.

The phrase 'You'll just have to manage' and the familiar 'coping syndrome' betray attitudes on the part of the manager and the managed which the profession should not be proud of.

Efficient managers will realise that frequent consultation with their staff on handling problems and strong support in obtaining the necessary help to overcome problems will make for a less weary and therefore less vulnerable work force.

Communication Systems

While it is in the daily nursing record that particular hazards or difficulties must be noted, two other professional communication systems should be utilised in the oral handover and in reporting to management.

An Oral Handover

An oral handover of information between members of the caring team may take place formally at the nursing report or the doctors' round, and informally at any time. Much *ad hoc* information emerges at these times, and it is very important that all care staff who are on duty should be present at the nursing report, and that the nurse allocated to the care of a particular patient should be present at the ward round when that patient is seen, and should record any changes in care agreed. In specialist rehabilitation units the presence of the physiotherapist at the nursing report has been found to be helpful.

An expanded communication system of this kind will enable the team to keep the doctor informed as to what can be realistically expected from the patient and any hazards to the nursing staff which his request for mobilisation might incur; and will enable the nurses and paramedical staff to be consistent in their approach to the patient, and make safe decisions about, for example, when hoist use should be reduced or withdrawn, or whether he is yet ready to attempt standing, etc. Team decisions can also be made about how many nurses are required to attend to the patient, what equipment should be used and the degree of trained staff supervision required. These decisions can then be written into the Care Plan.

Oral handovers with all carers present will also facilitate two way information between the people who are performing most of the handling tasks, i.e. the health care assistants and the trained personnel who may be away from the bedside more than they would wish. Health care assistants must always tell the nurse in charge immediately about any handling difficulty encountered, and make an entry in the nursing record.

Reports for Management

If a nurse is faced with an obvious handling hazard she should not attempt to move the patient, except in a life threatening situation, but should report the hazard to her line manager immediately. If a difficulty with handling is unresolved, despite oral reports, it is advisable for the nurse to put her concern in writing.

It is likewise recommended that employing authorities should have written policies on safe practice when handling patients, and that where specialised practice is required, e.g. for the handling of patients who have had strokes, spinal operations, hip replacements, or for handling of equipment in the operating theatre, then a local written procedure should be agreed.

Nurse managers have a responsibility to obtain the resources required for safe patient-handling in their units, and if their budgets are insufficient for the necessary expenditure, they will need to make a case to the health authority or trust administrator for additional provision. A report should be written detailing the prevailing hazards, the degree of risk to staff and the resources required to reduce the risk. Costings should be included. If an increase in staff allocated to the ward or community team is involved, the case will need to be very precisely stated in terms of risk to staff, and dependency levels of patients described in detail; instances where adequate provision of equipment, such as hoists, could reduce the need for extra staff should be pointed out.

Injury and Accident Investigation

The principles to be observed when investigating patient-handling injuries are set out in Chapter 5. The investigation must be prompt: and the onus is initially on the injured person to report and, as soon as reported, on management to set the investigation in motion. Investigation requires trained personnel. It must include information on the nature of the injury, for one of the first essentials is to establish the relationship between events complained of and the outcome in terms of the injury suffered: the extent to which the injury was work-related and the extent to which the injury should have been foreseen and prevented.

It is now a relatively simple matter to record injury data using the type of accident-models described on page 31, on computer files. An adequate form of initial investigation need take only 5-10 minutes in experienced hands. The data can then be stored and analysed to identify the main sources of risk: e.g.

whether the risks focus on individual patients, types of ward, lifting environments or on individual lifters and handlers. It is on this type of information that prevention can be based. The last two questions to be answered in any injury investigation are 'how could it have been avoided?' and 'what action is now needed?'.

Standards and Safety Audits

The Royal College of Nursing has introduced standards for quality assurance under the acronym 'DYSSY', Dynamic Standard Setting System. They serve to implement and extend Health Authority policies. The standard begins with the 'structure criteria' or items of service which enable the system to function. It is followed by the 'process criteria' which define the means to deliver the standard. It is completed by 'outcome criteria' to assess the achievements. Each employing authority will set standards to suit local conditions: thus standards will necessarily vary. The following text therefore addresses the broad definition of a policy on patient-handling: applicable to health authorities, local authority social services and privately run establishments for the care of sick and disabled people.

Although the development of patient-handling policies and standards follows the recommendations of the Health Services Advisory Committee (1984), few Employing Authorities have yet drawn up the necessary documents. An exception is Lewisham and North Southwark Health Authority (Guy's Lewisham and Optimum Trusts) and their *Code of Practice for Safe Patient Movement and Manual Handling of Loads* and the *Guidance Booklet* published in 1988*. Included in the policy is a 'movement hazard code' with its 'maximum weight units' which is incorporated in the individual's plan of care. A nurse tutor was appointed by the continuing education department. An extensive training programme for the training of 'trainers' was commenced. To monitor the working practices of nurses and the number of back injuries reported a yearly 'safety audit' was devised. This audit is used also to evaluate the training given, the working environment and its ergonomics.

The value of such a code of practice depends on the actions that are taken. One of the general benefits is educational, a better understanding of the problems. Another is the improved chain of communication. The need, for example, for a mobile hoist is recognised and acted upon promptly: so reducing foreseeable risks and increasing the efficiency of ward staff. Audit results can be incorporated into a quality assurance programme as, for example, the topic to be addressed by a 'quality circle'.

The development of a code of practice does not, and this must be emphasised, depend simply on writing it

and distributing copies to the members of a safety committee. The framework of communication and decision-making must also be established; with administrative channels kept open. It requires a wholehearted commitment from the highest levels of management, combined with the active cooperation of all the departments. Those who are charged with the development and enforcement of the code of practice must be vested with the necessary authority.

The policy is therefore the responsibility of management. It must carry the *imprimatur* of the governing body. Those who are charged with the duty of implementing the policy can be confident of doing so with the full authority of the governing body. Their first duty, or of the individual on the said body responsible for health and safety, is to write the policy: a policy that will impose duties and responsibilities on unit managers and others who may be answerable directly to the governing body. It will be drawn up to satisfy the following requirements:

The design of, and equipment for, patient-handling environments:
- when planning new buildings and accommodation;
- when refurbishing existing accommodation;
- when making *ad hoc* improvements to existing accommodation;
- in the selection of furniture and fittings.

The assessment of the patient-handling needs of individual patients/residents/clients:
- when the initial request for admission to the hospital, home or residence is made;
- when the individual Care Plan is drawn up on admission and at intervals dictated by progress;
- preparation of individual 'hazard' codes (patient's dependency, the environment and the methods of movement or transfer).

Assessment of other manual handling tasks

Selection and provision of hoists and other patient-handling or manual handling equipment

Accident reporting and investigation:
- date, time, site and witnesses to injury;
- task at the material time (including name and weight of patient involved) and description of objects associated with the accident or injury;
- nature of injury and clinical outcome;
- preventive action taken.

Annual or quarterly safety audit

Identification of high-risk problems:
- patients in Accident & Emergency, and in intensive care;
- the heavy, dependent patient;
- the aggressive or resistant patient;
- the unsafe environment.

---

* Available from The Nightingale and Guy's College of Health Continuing Education Dept, Lewisham Hospital, Lewisham High Street, London SE13 6LH.

Selection of Nurses/Carers for highrisk tasks

Education and training programme:
- unit managers, occupational health and safety staff, tutors;
- nursing officers, officers-in-charge, ward sisters, supervisors;
- others.

External consultation:
- ergonomics (The Professional Register of The Ergonomics Society);
- occupational therapy (The College of Occupational Therapists);
- physiotherapy (The Chartered Society of Physiotherapy and The Association of Chartered Physiotherapists in Occupational Health);
- other (including manufacturers, architects etc).

Assessment of Outcome.

The details and content of policy and the terms of each standard under each of these headings will vary with every employing authority, with the services they offer, with their management structure, with the size of their component units and with the professional resources available to them. Many organisations, though with the primary duty of nursing or domestic care for the sick and disabled, will have other employees exposed to manual handling risks: indeed to a variety of different occupational hazards. Clearly their safety policies concerning patient-handling must blend efficiently with other safety needs. Nonetheless the heart of any policy is derived from the collective and individual needs of the patients, residents or clients for whom the organisation exists: hence the emphasis on assessment, and allocation of functions, focused on the Care Plan.

The outcome of policy can be assessed epidemiologically, for example in terms of injuries or sickness absence from musculoskeletal disorders amongst the handlers, or by job-turnover. It can be assessed by studying the occurrence of accidents or work-stoppages associated with patient-handling. In continuing care wards, the effect of the policy can be assessed from changes in the dependency of patients, or in staffing requirements. Such policies or standards should ultimately show cost-benefits.

Training in Patient-handling (Ergonomics and Handling Skill)

Training is a requirement under statute law but the content and aims of training have never had much official consideration. Most of what is known and understood about training in manual handling is derived from industry and there is little or no evidence of its potential value. Fortunately, the benefits of training in manual handling have been demonstrated more with respect to patients and disabled people than to handling problems in industry.

First, it has been shown that education and training for student nurses, including basic biomechanics and ergonomics plus practical instruction in patient-handling skills, has led to improvement in the selection of handling method and its performance (Troup & Rauhala 1987). Secondly, Takala & Kukkonen (1987) reported that where 'on the job' training was provided, the use of mechanical lifting equipment was higher and stooped and twisted postures were less frequent. And the students who were best skilled in the selection and performance of handling technique were the least likely, on follow-up, to suffer back injuries (Videman et al. 1989). These studies, albeit limited epidemiologically, differ in both design and results from industrial studies of lifting-training in that they embody ergonomic features as well as an emphasis on physical skill.

The ground-rules for training in patient-handling remain the same:

- The first candidates for training are those in authority: unit managers, nursing officers, occupational health and safety staff, tutors, ward charge nurses/sisters, officers-in-charge. It could be deemed negligent to expose a junior or unqualified employee to work under the supervision of a senior employee who was ignorant or unaware of the principles of safe patient-handling.

- The training of learner handlers should not be confined to a classroom nor to a simulated environment (say in the practical room of a school of nursing) except when initially demonstrating techniques or when the learner adopts the role of patient. It must be provided at the place of work under experienced supervision. The training can only be said to be complete when the learner is confident, reliable and skilled in selecting and performing the appropriate range of techniques of patient-handling.

- A training technique which can be recommended is that of encouraging the learners to act as instructor, rehearsing aloud to their peers, what they have been taught.

The content of training will vary according to local needs and to the responsibility or authority of the trainees. A first essential is for the instructors to observe the current handling practice in the trainees' place of work: this is particularly necessary in the smaller units such as homes for the elderly. And it is unsafe to assume that the system of work during day shifts is a reliable mirror of what happens at night. But the basic pattern remains the same and should be planned under the following headings.

Warnings of Unsafe Handling Practices

Beginning with statutory requirements, the first duty may be to warn employers and employees of the risk of unsafe lifting and handling practices. They include (and here the use of the word 'lifting' is taken to encompass any manual force exertion while lifting, supporting, carrying, pushing or pulling):

lifting unnecessarily

lifting patients bodily

vertical lifting of loads in front of or to one side of the knees

prolonged lifting or holding

lifting in unstable postures

overestimation of lifting strength

failure to co-ordinate the action of two or more lifters.

Three examples of unsafe lifting practices have been given by way of additional warning in Chapter 5.

Assessment of the Patient

To begin with, handlers must learn to understand the practical significance of the warning not to lift unnecessarily. Partly out of goodwill and compassion, there is a tendency to save patients from having to shift for themselves. And paradoxically, patients are liable to be heaved from pillar to post simply to conform to some regime of management without giving them the chance to help themselves. In either case it is bad policy, it is bad for the patients and unnecessary. It stems from failure to assess the needs of the individual patient and failure to select the best solution to the problem of movement or transfer: such failures constitute bad management.

The assessment of the patient and disabled person is therefore at the forefront of training. At one extreme, patients may be unconscious and wholly dependent, while at the other are patients who are fully independent. Between these extremes there are stages of dependence or independence which can be assessed, say, on a scale of 1 to 6. But this is to beg an important question: to what extent can patients or disabled people be taught and equipped to become independent? Training should therefore offer guidance on how to assess the immediate and predicted needs and how to draw up or modify the Care Plan. In some cases, further assessment may be required from a physiotherapist, an occupational therapist or, perhaps, the community psychiatrist.

Allocation of Functions

This is a technical term from ergonomics: it poses the twin questions of what has to be done for the patient and what is the best way of doing it. In the case of patient-transfer, does the patient require assistance? Is this best provided, say, by a hoist? If not, how many handlers will be needed? And what handling equipment will be have to be used?

Take for example, an elderly-care ward and a patient who is being rehabilitated and encouraged to become more mobile. He is at present able to get about very slowly with a walking frame but with support from the nurse/carer. The need is to micturate. The options are to walk to the toilet, to be taken to the toilet in a wheelchair or for the curtains to be drawn and a commode brought to the bedside. The choice, of course, depends partly on the urgency of micturition and the solution may well be to take the patient to the toilet in a wheelchair and use the walking frame on the way back. Thus the problem begins with understanding the patient's needs, selecting the appropriate furniture and equipment; and then choosing the most efficient and comfortable method: in other words, the allocation of functions as between the patient, the handlers and mechanical handling equipment. This is the practical application of ergonomics: patient/handler ergonomics.

Assessment of the Handling Environment

The first question for the trainee to learn to answer is whether the environment is safe for handling. This is a matter of 'good housekeeping' and a fundamental lesson in safety (Saari 1987). The next question concerns architectural matters: in particular the space, the room for manoeuvre: if the toilet is too small to allow the direct transfer of a patient from wheelchair to WC, what are the alternatives? Then what other constraints are there on the proposed movements e.g. traction apparatus, drains or IV drips?

On the question of furniture and handling equipment, the trainee's critical faculties should be developed. Here it may be fruitful to refer to one or more of the publications in the series entitled *Equipment for Disabled People* from Oxfordshire Health Authority or to *Information Services* from the Disabled Living Foundation.

Assessment of the Handler

All potential handlers should be aware of their own handling or lifting capacities and those of their colleagues. Each should know the extent to which the other can be relied upon. Whether at a simple perceptual level or at the formalities of health screening, the individual criteria for assessing handling capacity are the same:

- Age
- Height, weight and lean body mass
- History of back trouble
- Occupational experience of manual handling
- Physical learning ability
- Patient-handling repertoire
- Gender
- Awareness of handling capacity.

Experience should teach people how much they can safely handle but this is not always to be relied upon. The recruit or learner must be watched and any sign of undue effort checked. But no-one's handling capacity is constant: it will vary with the time of day and everyone should beware of the effects of fatigue towards the end of the shift.

Instruction in Patient-handling Techniques

Having considered the purpose of the patient-handling task and assessed the patient, the handling environment and the handling capacity of the handlers, the technique can be selected. Here the instructor's task is to introduce the range of techniques from which the choice can be made. When the instruction programme is drawn up, the class should be divided into groups small enough to allow a handling trainer to supervise each nurse closely during practice.

Hoists and Mechanical Handling Equipment

Trainee handlers should first be introduced to the operation of hoists and the fittings and equipment that go with them. The message is that they are, or should be, labour-efficient. But here the instructor must beware lest the training is not put into practical use, routinely, in the ward or in the residence. The explanations for this failure are legion, though all should be investigated. One reason is that no hoists, or too few, are provided; the second is that either the wrong hoist has been chosen or the wrong fittings are to go with it e.g. a mobile hoist with only a plastic bath seat and no sling or other attachments suitable for patients with limited postural control; the third excuse is that it is out of order; and a fourth – a symptom of

nursing incompetence – is that the patients do not like it. In addition to conversancy with hoists, the trainee handler must become familiar with other mechanical aids to the movement, transfer and support of patients: not the items of equipment and the techniques for using them in isolation but in relation to the furniture, the equipment and the environment in which the handling is called for: hence the importance of providing the training at the work place and not in the classroom.

Manipulating the Handling Environment

Trainees should be taught the extent to which they can vary and improve the handling environment. Height-adjustment of the bed, placement of a wheelchair or commode, has to be taught in relation to the transfer technique that is chosen. The same applies to any preliminary movements required of or for the patient.

Manual Techniques

The natural athlete is a rare creature and the instructor must assume, to begin with, that the body awareness of the learner handlers is nil. The proper placement of the feet does not come naturally: it may have to be learnt. And instructors should have eyes like hawks. When learners find a technique to be less than comfortable, the most likely reason is that they are standing in the wrong place. For the instructor, practical instruction is often a 'hands-on' process; but remember that if you are lifting with the trainee in the course of instruction, you cannot always see what she is doing.

PART II.
PRINCIPLES
OF PATIENT-
HANDLING

Chapter 8 Promoting Patient Independence

Introduction

The primary objective when handling patients is to facilitate independent movement, and the nurse should help as little as possible. Weak or disabled people tend to forget their normal movement patterns and the nurse's task may be simply to remind them. The learner's introduction to patient-handling should include a reminder of basic human movement in which they analyse their own movements when sitting up in bed, getting out of bed, sitting down, standing up, etc., in order to establish some basic preliminaries in assisting patients.

Principles of Normal Movement

Sitting further back in the bed
1. Sit and lean forward.
2. Both hands palm down on bed behind buttocks, facing in.
3. One knee flexed.
4. Move bottom back by pushing on heel and hands.

Sitting on side of bed
1. Roll to one side then push up on hand and elbow nearest top of bed into sitting position and dangle feet over side of bed all in one movement.

Standing up from a chair
1. Draw feet back near to chair base, feet slightly apart one foot a little in front of the other.
2. Lean forward 'Nose over toes'.
3. Hands on arm rests.
4. Push up from hands on to feet.

Sitting down
1. With one foot behind the other and with back to the chair, feel the edges of the chair on back of legs. Flex the hips and grasp one or both arm rests.

2. Lower body-weight, pushing bottom right to the back of the chair.
3. Raise shoulders and then relax them for greater comfort.
4. Release skin tension under thighs.

Sitting further back in the chair if you have 'slumped' is a combination of the standing up and sitting down movements.

Getting up from the floor (first option for the fallen patient)
1. From flat on his back to side lying and then onto hands and knees.
2. Chair positioned alongside. Put nearside hand on seat or arm of chair, raise outside knee so that foot is flat on floor and pushing up on hand and foot raise bottom onto chair.

Turning over in bed
1. Roll onto back.
2. Shift trunk and shoulders, then bottom (see Bridging) back into the middle of the bed.
3. Turn head in direction of movement and lay outside arm over body.
4. Flex one or both knees and roll over, pushing bottom further through if necessary, to maintain position.

Bridging (Enables nurse to insert bed-pan or pull up undergarments)
1. Patient lying on his back, both knees flexed and feet flat on bed.
2. With forearms and hands (palm downwards, facing inwards) flat on bed, push down on hands and feet in order to raise bottom.

Moving to front of chair, prior to standing.
1. Patient leans forward and raises first one buttock and then the other to rock himself to the front of the chair.
2. Side rocking can also be used to enable the nurse to ease pants/trousers up or down.

Even though the patient may not be able to achieve these movements independently they should form the basis of any assistance given, and will often remove the need for a total lift. It is essential therefore that the nurse's action does not undermine the patient's own efforts.

As well as normal movement, patients' usual ways of moving should be considered. They may have found a way of moving over months or years of disability, which though unorthodox is successful, and the nurse should be ready to go along with it, as long as it is not stressful to either the nurse or the patient.

For the range of equipment for use by patients to maintain their independence, see Chapters 10-15.

Approach to Movement

A cardinal rule of skilled patient-handling is to move **with** the patient as far as possible, and not against him. For many patients an invitation to move, with assistance, will obtain a more positive response from the patient than being told that he is to be lifted, in which case he may stiffen himself in readiness for this alarming procedure, or else give up any notion of contributing himself. But the helpless patient, who cannot contribute in any way, will need to be helped to relax before he is moved.

The Neuromuscular Approach

This approach defines an efficient movement as "one which achieves it's objectives with the minimum of muscle effort and cumulative strain" (Vasey & Crozier 1982).

The approach recognises that repeated sustained contraction of muscle tissue causes a reduction in oxygen supply and predisposes towards loss of the natural elasticity of these structures leading to fatigue, strain and potential injury. Habitual top-heavy patterns of movement (stoop lifting etc.) are replaced by efficient patterns and applied in all areas of the subject's life – occupational, recreational and social.

Crozier teaches that a Conditioning and Patterning programme is an essential part of the whole re-education process which in the first instance deals with the mal-adaption of tissue due to top-heavy movement and secondly teaches a new pattern of movement to be applied to all basic actions (lifting, pushing, pulling, turning and reaching).

The principles which emerge:

- incorporate anatomical, physiological and physical principles;

- when applied, facilitate the recruitment of all available forces for any movement; muscle force being employed last and least;

- when applied, reduce the stiffening of tissue caused by any top-heavy movement; which in turn reduces cumulative strain and potential fatigue and injury.

If specifically considering the basic action of lifting, the recommended sequence would be:

- Relax, or let gravity unlock both knees.

- Move one foot in the direction of intended movement, or in the direction the operator is likely to fall.

- The first two steps above, now allow the back to relax in order to:

- Apply the hands as far under the load as is possible or feasible.

- The effort of the lift is now made by leading upward with the head to bring the vertebral column back to it's safest position.

Posture of the Nurse when Handling

Feet

The position of the feet is the secret of safe handling. If you are lifting within the area between your feet, you should be safe. If you lift outside this base you become unstable. Feet should therefore be apart and one in front of the other, balanced for the weight of the patient and the direction of movement. One foot must be close to the patient to take his weight at the beginning of the transfer, the other in the direction of movement and ready for where the patient's weight is to be transferred. Another reason for good foot placement is that it enables you to cope safely with an unexpected movement or the collapse or fall of the patient.

Knees

Use your knees. Lifting with your knees straight stiffens the whole lower limb, including the hip joint. It interferes with foot placement and thus restricts your lifting base. Moreover it prevents you from making use of the quadricep muscles to aid the lift. Therefore unlock your knees a little at the start of the lift and straighten them when actually lifting.

Never lift in front of the knees as this entails lifting at arms' length and never lift to one side of the knees as this involves twisting the spine. Do not hesitate to place one knee on the bed if this brings you closer to the patient.

When transferring a disabled patient the nurse can keep control of his movement and maintain his stability by pressing the inside of her knees against the outer side of his knees, but care should be taken not to upset his natural balance or prevent him moving his feet if he is able to.

Hands

The comfort of the patient, the avoidance of tender and painful areas and the sureness of the handlers' hold are the main criteria. The actual hold chosen depends on the type of transfer, on the way in which the patient can be parcelled and supported. It should give the maximal control of the posture and movements of the patient. Thus when grasping the patient's elbows they must be held firmly against his chest to prevent uncontrolled abduction at the shoulder; or when holding under the thigh, the hand should be close enough to the buttock to prevent unexpected hip flexion.

Anything which can be used as a handle is an advantage: a patient's belt for example. Patients' arms and legs are **NOT** handles. Plaster casts and splints can readily have handles incorporated to simplify the handling problems of moving and turning the patient. (See "Holds" page 69 for further comments).

Head and Back

Two common aphorisms of body movement are:

'The back should be kept as naturally erect as possible'

'Where the head goes, the trunk will follow'

These are aphorisms of body movement which those who handle loads, whether human or objects, need to build into their movement patterns. It is desirable but not always possible, that the back should be upright when lifting or carrying, or equally when maintaining a position, as for example when holding a patient's leg up for plastering. Leaning forward and holding that posture even as much as ten degrees adds measurably to the load on the vertebral column. But there is nothing wrong with bending the back to take hold of a load, provided the knees are unlocked and the feet positioned as described above. Indeed if the back is kept self-consciously straight right up to the moment when hands touch the ground, as for example when helping to lift a box off the floor, balance will be jeopardized and the average quadricep muscles may not be strong enough to lift the load from that level, so the back then 'jack-knives' out of control. On the other hand there is everything wrong with actually **lifting** the load with the back in flexion. This is where the head plays a vital part in protecting the spine: raising the head brings the lumbar curve back into the spine (lordosis), thus safeguarding it from the extreme flexion which can damage the disc.

Therefore as the load is taken up, the head should always be raised, and throughout the lift the load should be held as close to the body as possible.

The spine is also vulnerable when it is either rotated or bent sideways. **The position of the feet is the key factor in avoiding this.** Whenever a nurse's back is seen to be bent or twisted during a patient-transfer, almost invariably it is because her initial foot placement was faulty.

In addition to the posture of the back in terms of avoiding undue bending and twisting, it is essential to maintain a muscular control. Hollis (1991) recommends "dynamic abdominal bracing" in which the lower abdomen is flattened and braced upwards, but without hindering respiration in any way. Bracing is easily learned and "is an essential prerequisite of maintaining correct posture during a lift".

When lifting with one arm, the free hand should be used to stabilise the trunk and thus the posture of the back. It can be placed on the bed, as in the Shoulder Lift in which it is used as a strut to offload the spine and in which the active elbow extension actually aids in the lift. It can be placed on a table to give similar support or if there is nothing else to use when lifting with one arm, the free hand or forearm can be supported on the knee or thigh.

The principle of keeping the spine upright applies particularly to nursing procedures which do not necessarily involve lifting. There are innumerable jobs in which the nurse is bent over the patient for long periods and in which the spine is subjected to the cumulative effects of postural stress. This can be avoided or mitigated by adjusting the height of the bed, using the free hand to support the back, sitting on a stool etc (see Figures 13-16). Exposure to prolonged postural stress may precipitate a back injury.

In order to avoid any rotation of the spine at all when lifting with a knee on the bed, the helper's foot should also be right on the bed, and therefore a paper towel should be placed under it, or the shoe removed; possibly bootees as worn in theatre could be used. It is anticipated that if nurses follow the recommended practice of lifting manually only when it is absolutely unavoidable, these occasions will be so rare as to make this extra precaution taken in the interests of hygiene quite feasible.

The Position of the Patient

The patient should always be manoeuvred into an optimal position before the lift. Lifting strength is generally greatest when lifting with the hands at mid-thigh to hip-height; and the height of the bed or trolley should be adjusted accordingly. But when a patient who can take some weight on his legs is to be moved from his bed, the bed should be lowered until his feet can rest flat on the floor.

The more closely the line of weight of the patient's body can be aligned to the spine of the handler, the less the stress. The patient must be made into as compact a parcel as possible and his posture and movements controlled throughout the transfer. A nurse should beware of moving an unco-operative or struggling patient alone.

When a patient is expected to take only a little of his own weight the chair or commode to which he is being moved should be positioned so that he only has to turn 90° rather than 180° and his feet should be turned towards the finishing position before the transfer begins, in order to minimise any foot drag which may occur. He should be helped to the edge of the bed or chair before the transfer begins; this will enable him to get his weight over his feet more easily, and the nurse to avoid lifting at arm's length.

The Use of Body-weight

Using body-weight to take the effort out of manual work is a skill which has to be learnt and it needs a sense of timing and the understanding and cooperation of the patient. But once the skill is acquired, handling not only looks easier, it feels easier both for the nurse and the patient.

The principle is that if a body is moving it has momentum and thus kinetic energy. This can be used for a number of, but by no means all, handling tasks. Body-weight can be used in two ways to assist patient-transfers. One is by the nurse using her own body-weight and the principle of 'counterbalance'. The other is by means of the 'rocking principle'.

The use of counterbalance can be helpful when

raising a patient into a standing position. As the patient starts to come up so the helper lets her weight drop backwards to counterbalance and facilitate this action. But these skills have to be learnt. They need a sense of rhythm and timing and they need the understanding and co-operation of the patient.

In the 'rocking' techniques, kinetic energy for the transfer is developed for both nurse and patient. Many patients have learned how to do it for themselves. They rock themselves rhythmically backwards and forwards in the chair to build up the momentum or kinetic energy they need to stand-up. Using the same principle, a nurse can move a patient with minimal effort.

The 'rocking lifts' are for patients who can co-operate and are able to control their head and arm position. In effect their co-operation is mainly passive as they do not have to make any active effort. In the event that a patient resists the rocking, the nurse is immediately aware and can then take steps to overcome the difficulty.

There are two main applications for the 'rocking lifts'. One is for standing a patient up from a seated position: either preparatory for walking or when transferring from one seated position to another with the patient in an intermediate standing position. In the latter case, the patient is brought upright and supported while he is then turned into the position ready to sit down. The second application is for the 'rocking pivot transfer': a horizontal transfer of the patient direct from one seated position to another through some 90°. In this type of transfer the patient's feet remain on the floor and he remains in his sitting posture while 'in flight'. If necessary, say for a patient with painful ankles, a turntable can be used under his feet. Most 'rocking pivot transfers' can be performed by one nurse but two-nurses may be needed for a heavier patient. The applications are illustrated in Chapter 13 (see Figures 66 and 67).

Teamwork and Commands

When two or more nurses are lifting together, the need for co-ordination and timing is absolute. One of the nurses must act as a leader. It is her job to call the orders so that the place she takes must give her the best overview for keeping an eye, not only on any equipment such as a drip, but also on the patient's face. She gives the orders but only when everyone, including the patient, is ready and has said so.

When the leader calls the order, it must not only be distinct, it should set the rhythm. Not a 'one, two three and lift if you feel like it' tone of voice but a clear and incisive 'ready, STEADY, **LIFT**'

The actual wording is immaterial, as long as it is unambiguous. Two useful alternatives which have been adopted in some areas are:

'Ready, BRACE, **LIFT**' which encourages the lifters to brace their abdominal muscles to protect their spines as they lift.

'And.....HEAD' which encourages the lifters to raise their heads and thus straighten their backs as they lift.

WARNING

Don't bodily lift a patient on your own.

Don't lift or handle at arms' length.

Don't fail to ask for help when you want it.

Never lift at arms' length or with your back twisted.

Watch your working posture.

Table 4

SUMMARY OF THE PRINCIPLES OF SAFE HANDLING

1. NEVER manually lift a patient unless you have to in an emergency to ensure their safety.

2. ASSESS the patient and find out about his special needs which may affect the method you use to move him.

3. EXPLAIN what you are going to do and obtain the cooperation and consent of the patient.

4. ALWAYS use APPROPRIATE HANDLING EQUIPMENT if it is available.

5. PREPARE the handling area and watch for all hazards.

6. Know your own LIFTING CAPACITY and that of your lifting partners.

7. Your FEET should be apart, with one foot pointing away from the other and slightly in front, and your weight balanced between them.

8. Take a comfortable HAND HOLD, using the palm or surface of your hand and fingers. Keep your elbows tucked in to the sides of your body and hold the patient's belt, a sheet or handling equipment rather than the patient's body.

9. Always lift TOWARDS yourself, never away from you. Always hold the patient as close as possible to you. Use your own body-weight to balance and move the patient.

10. Do not TWIST your trunk when lifting. Relax your knees and raise your head as you lift to maintain a naturally erect spine.

11. Use RHYTHM AND TIMING when lifting and do not jerk. Always use clear instructions "Ready – STEADY – **LIFT**". Check with your lifting partner and the patient before moving.

Chapter 10
Basic Handling Equipment

The Dependent Patient

This type of patient is unable to assist with the transfer and may cause additional difficulties in that he has no control over his muscle tone, thus presenting the lifting staff with a floppy and often uncontrollable load. In addition to the patient's dependency, he could well be under going treatment that involves bottles, drips and stands, as well as other attachments, which further complicate the transfer and render the manual lifting technique hazardous.

Adjustable Height Patient Trolley

Adjustable height patient trolleys are always to be preferred for work in areas where the dependent patient may be received, treated and rested. Apart from the assistance that a low height will give to the more capable patient to get on and off the trolley, the higher height will enable the nurse to work in a more upright posture. The height-adjustment will also enable the patient to be transferred on or off any other fixed surface for diagnostic or treatment activities. Where high fixed-height couches or trolleys are in use, then alternative methods of assisting patients on and off these trolleys must be sought.

There is a mobile trolley (Fig. 22) which has been designed to adjust in height and to lift the patient mechanically on and off treatment tables. This trolley has a top frame with removable sheets that can travel with the patient through from ambulance to the ward bed. The sheet is X-ray translucent and either travels with the ambulance crew, or is immediately available on admission to hospital. The patient, having been placed on it, need not be manually lifted again until he is less dependent. The trolley top frame is raised up at an angle, the trolley chassis approaches the patient on the sheet on a table, the frame is lowered around him and the sheet attached on to the frame locks. The frame can then be raised in an horizontal plane so that the patient clears the table. He can then be wheeled and transported to the next area. Once at his new destination, the frame is lowered on to the

bed, the sheet unlocked, the frame raised and the trolley removed. This system would have considerable advantages in a busy accident and emergency department where patients have to be moved between beds, trolleys and diagnostic or treatment areas such as X-ray, plaster rooms and theatre.

Fig 22 *The mobile trolley*

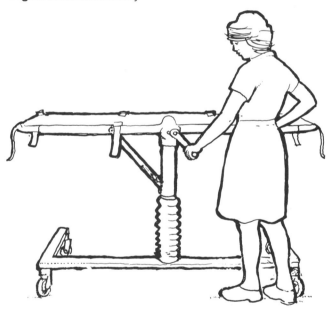

© NBPA

Stretcher Attachments on a Hoist

The Arjo-Mecanaids Ambulift hoist has a stretcher attachment which fits on its model D range (Fig. 23). This attachment has a metal frame which hooks on to the hoist spreader bar and the sling will support the whole body and also give bedpan access. For the dependent and yet conscious patient, a small pillow behind his head will ensure better comfort (if the patient's condition does not contra-indicate slight forward flexion of the neck). This may be a useful approach immediately following some surgical procedures where the patient may have to be nursed supine for 24 or 48 hours prior to being allowed into a

Fig 23 *Stretcher attachment for a hoist*

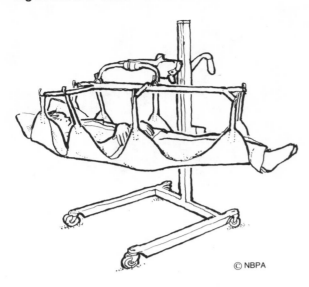

© NBPA

semi-sitting or more functional position. The use of this stretcher may also be useful where patients being prepared for theatre on the ward need to be transferred on to trolleys, or in the theatre itself where table to trolley to bed transfers are common.

Equipment To Move Supine Patient Between Bed and Trolley

The Use of Canvas Poles and Spreader Bars

This transfer is commonly used by porters and ambulance men. It is useful but can only be considered safe if the helper at the bedhead end can stand directly behind the patient's head to effect the transfer, without reaching across the bed to grasp the poles; this latter movement causes a dangerous stoop and rotation. If the bedhead cannot be removed to enable the helper to take up the correct starting position and there is no hoist or roller available, then it is preferable to loosen all the bed clothes and slide the patient across using one of the transfer aids or, provided there is no risk involved, by pulling on the undersheet. On no account should helpers lean across a trolley, or kneel on it, to lift a patient manually from the bed. Nurses and carers should beware of lifting on canvas and poles unless lifting height is optimised. Lifting at waist-height places an undue stress on the upper limbs. Use of canvas and poles is even more dangerous where the spreader bars are omitted.

Other Side to Side Transfer Products

Generally speaking the use of canvas and poles should be avoided. Other side to side transfer products are available to avoid the use of canvas and poles. Those of a more rigid design, such as the Scoop-stretcher, may still produce the postural difficulties caused by the canvas and poles method and care must be taken when lifting from a high fixed-height or where there are obstacles at the head and feet of the patient. On all side to side transfers the two surfaces need to be of the same height.

The Easy-slide (**Fig. 24a & b**) or the Handy-let are not rigid structures but more like a sleeping bag that is open both top and bottom. There is an outer cover for protection and an inner quilted section. The bag is the full length of a body and comes in a number of different widths. It is both comfortable for the patient to lie on and the two surfaces slide easily on each other. The patient lies on a sheet which one nurse uses to pull him into side lying, while the Easy-slide is edged beneath him. The second nurse on the far side of the surface on to which he is to be transferred, pulls the sheet towards her (not the Easy-slide), grasping it at the point of maximum weight of the patient i.e. the hips and shoulders. The patient slides easily over the two surfaces and there are no hard edges or protrusions which could harm the patient. The size and weight of the patient will determine the need for a third helper to pull.

The Easy-slide and the Handy-let are two soft, sliding items which are also available in a shorter form to assist with sliding the sitting patient up in the bed.

The Pat-slide, the Patient Roll Board and the Lateral Transfer Board are again similar, except that they are

Fig 24a *Sliding equipment transfer*

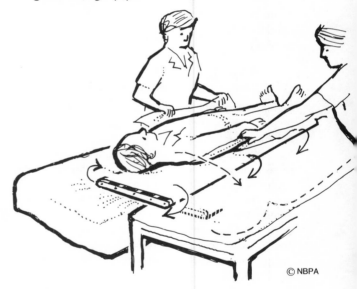

© NBPA

Fig 24b *A cross view*

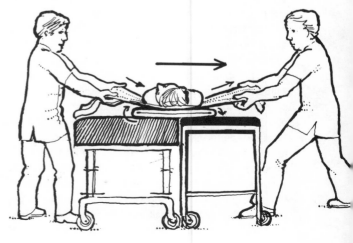

© NBPA

firm plastic boards which span the two transfer surfaces. The AIR-PAL is another type of supine transfer equipment which works on an inflated air bed. The compressed air sac is rolled beneath the patient and then inflated by a small electric pump. Once fully inflated, the patient can be moved around very easily since air is released through the base of the bed, enabling the patient's weight to be taken. It is similar to the principle of a hovercraft at sea.

There are commercially available Lifting Sheets which are strong, made of frictionless material and have handles along the sides of the sheet. These are best used for sliding the patient around the bed or from one surface to another. If they are to be used for lifting a patient, then the weight of the patient and the posture of the lifters must be assessed for any potential risk.

Hoists

There are three main categories of hoists:

- those fixed to a predetermined place
- those fixed to a track
- those which are mobile

Bath Hoists

The fixed-point hoists are mainly to be found in the bathroom where there is insufficient room to manoeuvre a mobile hoist. There are three types of bath hoists:

- those placed inside the bath and which only lift up and down from the base of the bath
- those sited outside the bath with a pillar mounting, so that a seat can be placed outside the bath for the transfer. The hoist can then be swung over the bath and lowered down: the seat may be detachable onto a wheeled chassis
- those where a socket on the floor of the bathroom will take the mast of a mobile hoist so that the same slings can be used. The patient is lifted in slings outside the bath, swung over and lowered into the base of the bath.

A description of the use of bath hoists will be found in the section on bathing a patient (see Chapter 15).

Electric Overhead Hoists

Electric Overhead Hoists (see Figure 78) are an important option where space is at a premium such as in a bathroom. Either a ceiling fixed track or a length of track on a moveable gantry may be used. The gantry is particularly useful in the community where the patient may be waiting for rehousing, is unable to make structural alterations to his home or has a prognosis indicating that short-term use of a hoist may be required. Electric overhead hoist design has recently improved so that many companies now offer cable free installations. In these, the power source is via rechargeable batteries which are topped

up whenever the hoist is not in use and 'parked' at a recharging point. This has enabled users to install overhead electric hoists, in ward bed bays and other such situations, without trailing cables.

In the community, these electric overhead hoists offer the possibility of the patient operating the hoist himself so providing an independent form of transfer. Recent changes in the way in which the Department of the Environment fund housing adaptations has meant that home owners are now subjected to a means-test. The reluctance of some patients to contribute financially to the installation of specialist equipment has meant that some community based staff are not able to use equipment best suited to their tasks. Where an alternative method is or becomes stressful, then a management decision must be made about the safe system of work available to community care staff.

Mobile Hoists

Mobile hoists (see Figure 72) may be subdivided into larger and smaller models. Both of these sizes are now available in either mechanically or electrically powered versions. While the hydraulic pumps and chain mechanisms of the mechanical hoists have been available for many years, the recent advance in small electric motors has enabled hoist manufacturers to offer an improved design for a relatively small additional cost. The electrically powered mobile hoist does offer a faster lift with less effort by the nurse. However, in choosing a model, check that there is not such an increase in the weight of the hoist that moving it from place to place (particularly in the community on a domestic carpet) becomes a heavy task.

With the emphasis on patients returning to their own homes, the smaller hoists might be suitable for both use on the ward and for training purposes as well as in the more confined space of domestic houses. This is particularly true when considering the rehabilitation or resettlement of elderly patients. Their handling assessment should be completed while they are in hospital so that on discharge home, or to a residential-care establishment, a safe system of handling can be implemented by all the care staff. If the same community hoist equipment is available on the ward, then the elderly person can become used to the equipment prior to discharge and thus ease the task of the community nurse.

Hoist Slings

Slings which give all round support to the body are needed for high dependency patients, but the design used must depend on both the patient's body shape, the degree of comfort and support which it gives and the purpose for which it is needed. Slings may be broadly divided into the following types of designs:

- hammock or divided leg design
- all-in-one design
- two or three piece slings

The use of a hoist and sling should ease the stress of handling. If a patient still has to be lifted on and off a sling, then probably the wrong design of sling has been chosen. Therefore, while it may be possible to roll the patient on to an all-in-one sling on the bed, the sling must remain in position as long as the patient is sitting on it after the transfer. It may be necessary to take precautionary measures, such as lining the sling with sheepskin, to prevent the development of pressure sores.

Hammock or Divided Leg Design. The hammock or divide leg sling (**Fig. 25**) can be positioned while the patient is sitting. The patient is supported and leans

Fig 25 *Hammock sling*

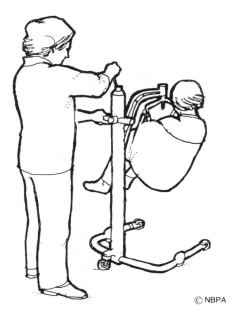

© NBPA

Fig 26 *Hammock sling*

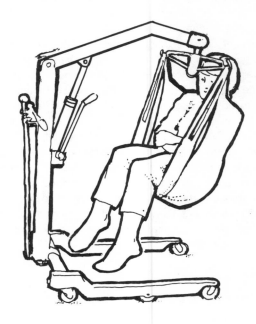

© NBPA

Fig 27 *Divided leg sling*

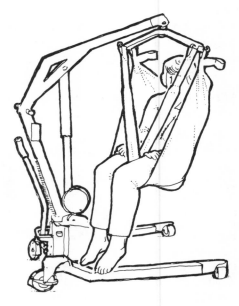

© NBPA

forward while the sling is pushed down the back of the chair so that the centre of the top of the sling is located at the patient's neck and the centre of the lower curved part is at the base of the patient's spine. The patient sits back in the chair, thus holding the back of the sling in position. The two leg pieces are pulled around, one to each side of each thigh. It will help if the patient is seated on a cushioned surface as the edge of the sling can be eased under the patient's buttocks if the nurse's fingers press the edge of the sling down and into the cushion. The leg pieces may then be attached in one of three different ways;

- each leg piece is crossed under both thighs and attached to the hoist spreader bar on the opposite side. This results in the legs being lifted together, which is both more comfortable and more dignified for the patient, (particularly for ladies wearing skirts). Where pressure between the knees may cause discomfort e.g. in inflamed knee joints, then a soft pad of sheepskin between the knees may relieve this, as might an alternative positioning of the leg pieces (**Fig.26**).

- the second method is to pass the leg pieces under each thigh and attach them to the spreader bar on the same side. This can be

uncomfortable for the patient with little muscle tone since the legs will abduct when lifted. However, it may provide easier access for cleaning while toiletting.

- the last method is to pass the leg piece under each thigh and fasten it to the opposite side so that the legs are suspended separately but they hang together when lifted. This may also be useful for cleaning after toiletting as the legs can be held apart (**Fig.27**).

All-in-one Design. The all-in-one design (**Fig. 28**) is most useful when the patient is in pain and does not wish to be handled manually. It is also useful where carers are themselves frail and find that the placing of slings causes them stress and concern. Where a transfer is to take place particularly in a confined

Fig 28 *All-in-one design*

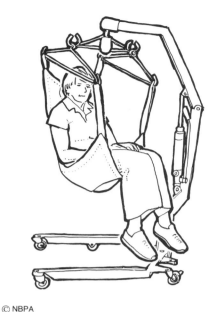

© NBPA

Fig 29 *Using an all-in-one sling in and out of a car*

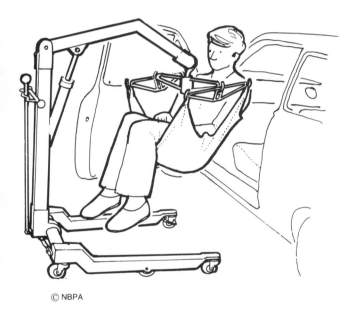

© NBPA

Fig 30 *Two or three piece sling*

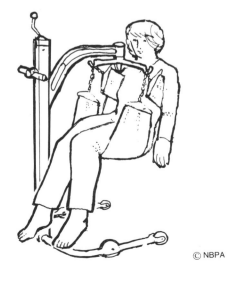

© NBPA

area, for example in and out of a car, then this sling can be left in place, thus avoiding the need for a carer to stoop and twist in order to place the sling around the patient (**Fig.29**).

This sling is used successfully with patients who have had a double leg amputation. The sling supports them safely and comfortably. Some adjustment to the length of the suspension straps may have to be made to compensate for the lack of leg weight and an altering of the patient's centre of gravity.

Two or Three Piece Slings (Fig. 30) Two or three piece slings need to be placed with care as there is a risk of jack-knifing if the thigh sling is not placed high enough under the hip joint. Another discomfort with these types of slings is the strain through the patient's axillae which is most uncomfortable for an arthritic shoulder joint.

Recently developed slings to assisst with the management of clothing while toiletting, are easy to use, and comfortable for the patient. The top sling often has a velcro fastened waist support to avoid or minimise the pressure under the axillae. The thigh piece is oftened stiffened to give support beneath the thighs.

In deciding which design of sling to use, several factors should be taken into account:

- how much support does the patient need?

- in what body position should the patient be transferred and what position gives the patient maximum comfort and functional position?

- is the carer capable of placing the slings quickly and correctly, or would a frail carer be better using an all-in-one sling which stays under the patient?

Developments by all manufacturers have improved sling design by eliminating the need for metal work and chain suspensions. This has assisted in both the laundering of slings and their quieter use which must comfort both the nurse and the more easily, confused or apprehensive patient.

Remember, as good practice, always match the sling and hoist, both should be from the same manufacturer. Several companies are now able to offer a made-to-measure service so that if they cannot provide a standard sling to meet the patient's needs, then they are able to design and make a 'special'. Indeed it is by requesting these different slings that a new design is often developed to be marketed more generaly for the benefit of all hoist users.

Choosing A Hoist

The following check list may assist in selecting the right type of hoist from an increasingly wide range:

- Consider all the transfers that currently take place. List where they occur and how often. For an individual patient in the community, think through all the transfers to be made during 24 hours. In a hospital environment, ask several staff to list every time they lift or handle a patient.

  From this list, stop and consider if all these transfers are necessary, or whether there is another way of performing the task. Can some of the transfers be eliminated? Are you seeking a hoist which will lift patients over twenty stone many times a day or a lighter model which will lift up to twenty stone fewer times? Are there any special hoist features such as a weighing scales or a self-operating facility which will assist the patients?

- Having selected the areas and patients involved in the transfers, focus on the environment in which the lifts take place. Space is often the controlling factor. How much space is there between beds; beside the toilet; in the passageways and through door widths? Are there any tight corners, steps, stairs or ramps to be negotiated?

From these two first considerations, it should be possible to short-list a number of hoists which will lift the weights required and which will work in the space available. Access may be required to a data base of currently available hoists such as that provided to subscribers of the Disabled Living Foundation's Information Service.

- Having obtained the data sheets for the shortlist of hoists, check out the measurements against the areas where the hoist is to be used.

- Next look at the range of slings and additional extra facilities which are offered with each hoist. If there is a wide variety of patients with varying disabilities and dependencies, then a range of slings to suit these differing needs is important.

REMEMBER: A chosen sling should be used on the hoist from the same manufacturer. **DO NOT** mix slings and hoists from different manufacturers.

- Once a short-list of products and slings has been made, ask for a demonstration, if possible in the area in which they are to be used. Does the product actually do what the nursing staff and patients want it to do?

- When the hoist and slings have been chosen and the order placed, consider how the full use of the hoist is to be implemented and arrange for any training sessions for users when the equipment is delivered.

- It is often helpful if a product can be left *in situ* for a few days prior to the order being placed so that all staff have a chance to see, try and comment on its suitability.

- Once the training has taken place, follow-up checks are required to confirm that the choice was a correct one and that the hoist has improved the safety of the handling tasks in that working area. This is particularly important in the community where a community nurse may not visit regularly once a hoist is introduced and other carers continue their tasks with the patient.

- Finally ensure that regular maintenance takes place. All hoists should be serviced at least once a year and BS 5827 outlines the type of inspection and maintenance required of all mobile patient lifters (BS 5827 (1979)). Records should be kept of all equipment outlining its purchase date, repairs and routine services.

In summary, hoists eliminate the need for manual lifting. They are comfortable for the patient. They can be operated by one nurse or carer or, in some instances, by the patient himself. They are therefore both safe and labour saving.

Walking or Handling Belts

Patients requiring the assistance of a nurse may have painful joints or be lacking a limb which makes it difficult for the nurse to decide where to place her hands to take some of the patient's weight. In many instances a Handling Belt worn by the patient will provide a comfortable handhold for the nurse without distress to the patient and enable the nurse to hold him securely while walking or transferring. A Handling or Walking Belt should be at least 2″ wide with an adjustable snap fastening. Some designs also have webbing handles stitched on the outside so that the nurse does not have to place her fingers against the patient's skin. The belt is passed around the patient's waist, snapped shut and pulled tightly to fit. This is particularly useful when the patient has no clothing on and may also be wet and slippery. Wide leather belts can also be conveniently used, but only over clothing. Handling Belts are recommended for helping patients who have had strokes because they minimise the risk of damage to a paralysed shoulder joint.

Turntables

Some patients who may have stiff or painful legs and ankles may find that their feet twist when being assisted from one sitting position to another: for example from the bed to commode or chair. There is a variety of turntables which come in a number of different diameters, surfaces, materials and weights. The patient is positioned and prepared for the transfer. The turntable is placed with his feet positioned centrally on the top surface and midway

Fig 31 *Use of turntable with handling belt*

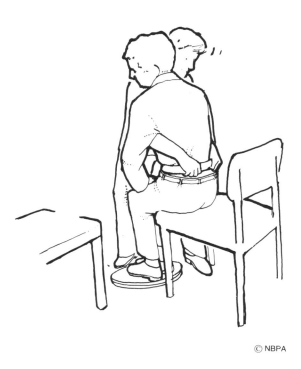

© NBPA

between the two transfer seats. The nurse immediately places one of her feet against the turntable to prevent it moving before everyone is ready. Some patients may feel the turntable move slightly, which causes anxiety about the possible instability of the transfer. The nurse positions herself in front of the patient and using a pelvic waist-band lift (or using a lifting belt) or a rocking lift, the patient is raised to his feet and moved through 90° to the next seat (**Fig. 31**). As the patient is raised, so the nurse slightly moves her foot to free the turntable which then turns so that the patient's feet are aligned as he sits again. This is not suitable for the confused patient; nor should it be left on the floor for staff or patients to step on accidentally.

Basic Handling Equipment for Use by the Patient

A variety of equipment is available which will offers the elderly frail person, or a person with a disability, a degree of independence; and will minimise the stress on the carer. Most will require the disabled person to have good balance and some strength in his arms. All these items are equally useful within a community or hospital environment since the tasks with which they seek to assist are those performed in either setting. It is wise to remember that a disabled person admitted to hospital may require to continue using his own independent transfer system, if he is not to lose abilities that he will again need on his discharge home.

Patient Hand-blocks

Hand-blocks can be used singly or as a pair (see

Figure 91). They are particularly used to enable the patient to raise himself off the mattress or to move up and down the bed. If he is using it on only one side, then the patient must be able to assist the nurse or relative by grasping the hand-block in his good hand and pushing with his stronger arm, while also pushing down on his stronger leg. The nurse positions herself on the patient's weaker side and either by using a Through-arm Lift or a modified Shoulder Lift, can ease and support the patient on his affected side.

Sliding or Transfer Boards

This is a smooth rectangular piece of wood which is bevelled at its narrower edges (see Figure 55). The patient with good upper limbs can place the board beneath his hips as he sits in the wheelchair and across on to the bed. He can then readily slide himself across to the adjacent surface. While this is a simple and easily transported aid, the furniture and surfaces for transfer must be of similar heights. This system is particularly useful for single or double lower limb amputees where the upper limb function is not significantly impaired. Apart from its use in and out of bed or other seated positions, it is widely used for car transfers to and from a wheelchair.

Car Transfers

First the car is parked with space on the passenger side, and the front passenger seat is moved back to create maximum leg room for the disabled passenger. The patient in his wheelchair is positioned by the opened passenger car door. The wheelchair's nearside arm is removed and the patient rests his feet on the door sill of the car. The transfer board is tucked beneath the patient's hips as he is gently supported to one side. This is much easier if the patient is seated on a wheelchair cushion since the board can be dug into the cushion's softer surface. The handler then goes around the car and kneels on the drivers seat facing the patient. It is helpful if the patient is wearing a lifting belt so that the handler has something strong to grasp. The handler braces herself with her left hand along the top of the passenger seat back while her right hand grasps the patient's belt. The patient can assist by bringing his weight forward and perhaps maintaining a good posture by propping himself upright on an opened car window ledge etc. At a clear given command, the handler pulls the patient towards her in a straight line and the patient will slide over and into the seat. His feet should also be correctly aligned since his feet were placed on the car sill prior to the transfer. With practice this is a comfortable and easy transfer requiring minimal equipment and avoids the need to manually adjust the patient back in the car seat

Recently, a design of transfer board has appeared which is curved in shape, rather like a 'banana'. These can be useful when transferring on to surfaces with fixed arms such as a favourite armchair or into a car with rally type supportive seats.

Trapeze Lift or Monkey-pole

Almost all hospital beds can be fitted with an overhead trapeze lift which will enable patients with good upper limbs to heave themselves up or turn over in bed. The patient should be taught to lift his pelvis from the bed in order that a bedpan can be slipped beneath him. This is called 'bridging' (see Figure 42) and can easily be achieved by the patient pulling on an overhead trapeze lift. The handle of the lift may need to be padded and should be adjusted to the correct height for each patient. Where this type of aid is used with a divan headboard, it should be securely fastened with a bracket to avoid the upright lift pole from moving while in use. If the nurse is assisting the patient while he is using a trapeze lift, care should be taken to avoid the patient swinging away from the nurse and thus putting the nurse in a position of postural stress. Fixed or free-standing lifting poles are also available for use with a divan or other bed at home and in the community.

Apart from use of the trapeze lift in hospital or the community, use may be made of small wall-fixed rails which can greatly assist the patient's ability to pull himself into a seated position. These are widely used in the community and a small rail beside the bed, or to ease getting on or off a stairlift seat will make the patient both safer and more independent.

Bed Ladder

This is a simple item of equipment which consists of two lengths of thin ropes between which are fastened a number of wooden cross pieces (the rungs of the ladder). The ends of the ropes are fastened to each of the bottom legs of the bed so that the rungs come within handhold reach of the patient. When the patient wants to turnover in bed or to sit up, he grasps the rungs of the 'ladder' and pulls it towards himself so taking some of the weight of his upper body and making it easier for him either to move himself or for the carer to assist him.

Beds

The design of beds will be discussed further in Chapter 12; however, it must not be forgotten that correct bed design not only assists the carer but may also make the patient independent. The bed mattress height is of prime importance when transferring a patient to and from bed. It should be as close to the height of the wheelchair or commode seat as possible. To achieve this correct height, there are a number of designs of bed leg sleeves which will raise the height of a low divan bed. Alternatively, it is possible to replace some divan bed castors with a wooden leg also with a castor. In this way the height of the bed is raised and the bed remains mobile for cleaning and for ease of access by the carer. Some beds are electrically controlled by the patient and he can alter the position from lying to sitting by adjusting the angles of the head and feet sections. This is extremely useful in the community where a patient can often change his position or relieve muscle spasms by altering his bed position automatically rather than having to wake a carer from her sleep at night.

Bed Back Rests

A wide variety of bed back rests is commercially available in metal, plastic or wood. There are also the padded armchair shapes which rest on the bed and sometimes provide pockets for patient's belongings. The 'V' shaped pillows have also been found to be useful where very elderly and frail patients have required a soft pillow to support them while sitting in a comfortable easy chair or in bed.

Bed Leg Lifter

One of the most frequent reasons for Home Care or Community Nursing Services being required to assist patients to bed at night is because the patient is unable to lift his legs into bed on his own. It is worth considering the several products which have been designed specifically for this task. Some have now been developed so that they are electrically controlled while others are designed to help those who have some movement but not enough strength. The patient places his feet on a board or platform at ground level as he sits on his bed. As he lies back against the pillows, so the feet are raised to be level with the mattress so that the patient can roll them sideways into the bed. Some patients may be able to achieve this by using a length of bandage or a scarf as a sling around their legs to lift them in one at a time.

Bathroom and Toilet

The bath board and seat (see Figure 75), together with a non-slip bath mat, are perhaps some of the first equipment items that disabled people will be introduced to. Their full use is described in Chapter 15, Washing and Bathing.

For disabled people in the community, using the toilet and showering can become an independent task with the provision of a self-propelling shower chair or sani-chair. Often an attendant operated chair is provided, that is one with four small castors, instead of one with two larger wheels that will allow the person to propel himself. The right choice and design will allow the patient to transfer from his bed to the chair, for him to move himself to the bathroom and wheel himself over to the toilet and then to push himself again into a flat access shower area to be washed. Thus the right choice of equipment alleviates the need for multiple transfers.

A refinement on shower sani-chairs is the elevating seat. This is useful for those patients who can walk slowly once they are on their feet but limited hip flexion makes it both difficult for the helper and painful for the patient. The provision of a lifting seat on the toilet/shower chair means that the patient can rise independently, rather than having the carer pull at a stiff and painful body.

Wheelchairs

Wheelchairs can either be bulk purchased for general use within a hospital or community loan service, or can be specifically prescribed through a district based wheelchair service for an individual patient. Now that the supply of individual wheelchairs is managed locally, each Health District will have its own organisation and budget. However, it is worth reviewing the features of wheelchair design in order that the right wheelchair can be provided either for the individual and his handling and transfer needs, or for general use by hospital patients many, of whom will have mobility and transfer difficulties.

The first consideration is the use to which the wheelchair will be put. The height and weight of the user will affect the structure of the model chosen. Most wheelchairs will carry people of up to fourteen stone, but above that weight a stronger chair frame will be required. For portering services in hospital, the prospect of handling and transporting patients of 25 – 35 stone must be considered, so that some strong wheelchairs will be required. The user's disability or general level of functioning will also affect the chair design. Those people with poor posture will require a more supportive wheelchair than provided by the transit chairs often used in hospital which have wide seats and open low arms. Is the patient to operate the wheelchair himself or will it be pushed by the attendant? Will the wheelchair be used indoors and outdoors and on what type of ground?

Types of Wheelchair

There are basically four types of wheelchair design.

Transit Chair

The Transit Chair is provided mainly for outdoors and has four smaller wheels. The patient cannot self-propel it and an attendant pushes it. Many of these transit chairs have fixed arms which make it difficult to transfer. The footrests usually swing up but may not always be removable. Some such chairs have foot-rests which allow the patient to stand on them safely without tipping the chair.

Self-propelling Wheelchair

The Self-propelling wheelchair has two larger wheels, usually at the back but could alternatively be in the front; the other two wheels being smaller castors. Many attendants find that this is an easier chair to push and to manoeuvre when going up and down ramps, steps and stairs. The weight of the patient can be rolled back on to the two larger rear wheels thus bringing the weight closer to the attendant and easier to control over rougher ground. Many patients prefer this type of wheelchair, since few are unable to move themselves a short distance by using the hand rims

on the larger wheels. Most of these wheelchairs have removable arms and footrests. The back of the wheelchair usually has two catches which when released allow the top half of the chair back to be lowered backwards. This moves the pushing handles down and out of the way of any handler who is assisting the patient from behind.

Electric Wheelchairs

Electric wheelchairs can either be patient or attendant operated. They can be designed for indoor use only, or indoor and outdoor use and for outdoor only. The attendant operated chairs are of benefit to those carers who may need such assistance in order to push a patient outdoors. Generally the local district wheelchair services only supply indoor electric models to patients although some are experimenting with indoor/outdoor models. Electric outdoor wheelchairs are only available through private purchase and much care must be taken over the choice of a suitable model. In handling terms, the points to consider usually focus around the need to transport the electric wheelchair from place to place. The ability to fold and lift it in and out of a car boot may be a key requisite. Most patients who use such wheelchairs have poor physical function and may be unable to assist with transfers. It is important also to check if armrests and footrests are removable for both side-ways transfers and for weight relief when transporting it. The camber of road and pavements, the height of kerbstones and slopes down to the gate are also important considerations.

Childrens' Wheelchairs and Buggies

Childrens' wheelchairs and buggies come in a large variety of shapes, sizes, colours and construction. Carers need to be taught how to handle children in and out of low buggies and to take preventitive measures when pushing such childrens' equipment for long periods. Many chairs are too low and carers find themselves walking and pushing a load in a stooped position. If a design of buggy cannot be found that suits their own height, then measures may have to be taken to plan a trip that involves stops and rests when the carer can stretch and relax in order to relieve the stress of continual stooping.

Wheelchair Features

The desirable features for a handler to look for on a wheelchair will include;

Footplates

Footplates that are adjustable in height and which swing and detach to create space for sideways transfers. Fixed footplates are a hazard and models which still have them should be withdrawn from use in institutions.

Armrests

Armrests that are easily removable but still have a safety catch to prevent accidental detachment. Some armrests are also adjustable in height so that the disabled person has his arms and shoulders supported in alignment. This may mean that the disabled person can take his weight through his upper arm by pushing through his elbows on the correctly adjusted armrest. This may be useful when placing a hoist sling around him.

Back Rests

Back rests that fold down allow the lifter to stand close to the patient without the obstruction of the pushing handles. There may be an extension headrest or other brace that has to be removed before the patient can be transferred in and out of his chair.

Wheels

Wheels may be large or small. The larger propelling wheels of a wheelchair may be an impediment when transferring sideways using a sliding or transfer board. Those disabled people who have used large front propelling wheels may present transfer difficulties as their abilities decline later in life.

Brakes

Brakes are important on all wheelchairs. The carer must ensure that the brakes are **ON** before starting any transfer manoeuvre. It is sometimes possible to add extension handles to brakes so that they can be easily reached without stooping by either the carer of the disabled person. The control box for an electric wheelchair also contains a braking system and any electric chair must also be switched OFF before any transfer is attempted.

Cushions

Cushions provide not only comfort and pressure relief but also enable a handler to insert hoist slings, transfer boards and other small handling equipment items beneath the patient's thigh or hip without causing discomfort. A thicker cushion can also be used to place the patient at a better height for a transfer. Back cushions and other specially designed forms can help alleviate the discomfort many disabled people feel while in their wheelchairs. If people feel comfortable and relaxed, then they co-operate and are able to assist the handler better.

Body Moulds

Body moulds are used by some children and adults who have little or no postural control of their own. These moulds are tailor-made for individual users and help to position the person in a way that enables them to function at the highest possible level. When a mould is to be prescribed and its use considered, there are several points that affect the design.

- If the user is to be a hoist user, then the mould must not be such a tight fit that a sling cannot be eased around them.

- If a shape is being prepared for a wheelchair mould, it is worth considering whether there are other uses for this type of support. A thinner plastic mould may be formed and mounted on a sani-chair frame. With a hole

cut out in the seat area, this can then be used as a very supportive toilet chair to push over the WC, and as a shower chair. This must alleviate some of the transfer and handling problems associated with these disabled people and the postural stress experienced by so many of their care staff.

- If transport in a car is to be considered, then the possibility of the disabled person staying in the mould must be a comfortable option. If a handle is incorporated on the top of the base board that supports the mould on the wheelchair seat, then it is possible to grasp this and use a transfer board for car transfers as described on page 61. The car safety strap will fit over the person in his mould, thus making him safe and comfortably secure for his journeys.

Weight of Wheelchairs

So often carers ask for a really lightweight wheelchair since they have developed low back pain from pushing and lifting wheelchairs, with or without their occupants, over a long period of time. The lighter wheelchairs generally do not stand up to daily use and the heavier weights of many adult disabled people. It may be better to ensure that all wheelchair users (including the carers) receive instructions on how the wheelchair is to be folded and lifted in and out of cars.

Lifting a Wheelchair In and Out of a Car

The best car boot for wheelchair carriage is the hatchback where the boot lid comes right down to the bumper. In cars where there is a high ledge to lift over, then there are difficulties in following the principles of safe handling. It is useful to carry a travelling rug, spare piece of old carpet or a rubber mat in the boot of the car so that this can be pulled forward and laid over the car rim and bumper to protect the paintwork. The brakes are applied and the empty wheelchair is folded by pulling up on the seat canvas. Both armrests and footrests are removed and placed in the boot at the sides. The back of the wheelchair is folded so that the handles are tucked in. The wheelchair is now a square shape and a more compact load. Some people find it helpful to put a luggage strap around the chair to provide a handle for lifting. The carer then grasps the chair on any upright and non-moving part and pulls the chair towards themselves. The load can now be held as close to the lifter as possible. The wheelchair is swung towards the lifter and pivoted on the lower edge on to the rim of the boot (hence the need for protection). Once the wheelchair is balanced there, the weight is taken from the lifter. The wheelchair is then tipped away from the lifter into the boot and manoeuvred until the boot will close. It is often easier to remove the parcel shelf in a boot and travel with the wheelchair in a more upright position than to try to lie it down flat on the boot floor. A black plastic bag on the boot floor will enable some loads to be pushed and pulled around the boot without lifting the weight while it is furthest from the handler.

If it is difficult to lift a wheelchair in and out of a car boot, several other options remain. The wheelchair can be folded as previously described and then rolled and rocked into the space between the driver's seat and the back seat. This is easiest in a two-door car. The front castors of the chair are rested on the car sill and the back section of the chair tipped up and rolled forward till the wheelchair rolls into place. The driver's seat can then be readjusted. Other options include the type of hoist that will hook the wheelchair up and lift it on to the roof in a specially designed compartment or will hook it on to the door adjacent to the driver. A further idea is to replace the car seat with a wheelchair seat so that the disabled person stays in his seat with no necessity for transfers, or he has a car or van specially designed to take him in his wheelchair by a ramped entry from behind.

For disabled people who are at work or who attend a regular venue, it may be possible to consider two wheelchairs, one at both venues to avoid the need to lift, carry or transport such a heavy and awkward item.

Where disabled people and/or children have to be transported by vehicles which are provided by Social Services, Education or Health Care agencies, then due regard to the design of this transport must be made. If people in wheelchairs have to be regularly transported then a tail lift must be supplied on the bus. It is not acceptable to allow any care staff to lift adults or children manually on and off buses in a stooped and awkward position. The roof height in the bus must allow an adult carer who is acting as an escort to stand upright. The seating arrangements must be flexible enough to allow wheelchairs to be fastened to the bus floor or for seats to sit those people who can transfer easily.

Commode Design

It is regrettable that commodes used both in hospital and the community are not always of a design that assists with the transfers of patients. It is often an item which is regarded as cheap and expendable while a short time spent considering what is needed may improve safety in handling for both staff and patients.

When purchasing a new supply of commodes, the patient's needs must come first. If the patients are adult or over eight stone in weight, dependent and non weight-bearing, then hoist use is indicated and the design of commode may be different to that required by an independent but disabled patient.

Equipment Information

In concluding this chapter, much emphasis must now be made on the fuller use of mechanical hoists and other handling equipment. Until now, few hospitals have been adequately equipped and thus few nurses are fully experienced in the use of mechanical lifting equipment.

Access to information about ranges of products is an important factor when spending valuable financial resources on equipment. The national network of Disabled Living Centres (see Appendix for addresses) offer a demonstration and information resource on all equipment associated with disability. Staff at these centres are experienced in evaluating products and assisting inquirers to select equipment most suited to their own and their patient's needs. Subscribers to the Information Service at the Disabled Living Foundation will also have access to product data to assist with purchasing decisions. Before deciding on the equipment which would help you best, be sure to have them demonstrated in your own workplace or in the patient's own home before placing an order.

PART III.
PATIENT-HANDLING PRACTICE

Chapter 11
Patient-handling

Preparation

There are a number of points to be remembered and acted upon before actually moving the patient. First, there is the general question of the purpose to be served by the move and the condition of the patient. Could he be helped to move himself? Could a mechanical aid be used? The handling technique can then be selected and the number of nurses who will be required can be assembled. When seeking a lifting partner, compatible heights and lifting capabilities should be taken into account. If an additional procedure is undertaken while the handling is taking place e.g. inserting a bedpan or guarding an injured limb, then an extra nurse will be required. There must be no doubt which of the nurses is to act as leader, explaining matters to the patient and giving the word of command; in some instances, the patient may be asked to give the word of command. Furniture must be moved to the most convenient position, all hazards removed, brakes applied on trolleys, beds and wheelchairs and the height of the bed adjusted where possible and the bed clothing made ready. Then, and not before, they are ready for the lift itself, for which the basic rules have been set out at the end of Chapter 9.

Holds

The way in which the helper takes up her hold on the patient will give him a strong message about her intentions and what is expected of him, and he will respond accordingly. For example, a frontal approach, or a pull may obtain a reflex pull in the opposite direction, as happens when the Drag Lift is used (see p.32). But standing at the side of the patient, in a co-operative rather than operative stance, or 'stroking' the patient in the direction of movement before actually taking up a hold is an approach more likely to trigger the required movement, and inspire confidence and a feeling of security. This is known as an 'indirect approach'.

Another important principle when obtaining a hold is to extend the hands and trunk further than necessary and then let the hands settle back into a palmar hold. In this way, body-weight rather than purely finger/

hand grasp is used to initiate movement of the load, and lifting strain is more widely and evenly distributed.

Holds for Use by One Nurse

These one-person holds are intended to support and move a patient who is able to give some assistance and to bear some of his own weight:

Elbow Lift Hold

This is useful for transferring in a confined space and easily carried out by a nurse who is tall enough to reach over the seated patient. She stands in front and to one side of the patient, with one foot beside him and the other in front blocking his knees. She should feel stable and able to move her weight freely from one foot to the other. She encourages or helps the patient to lean forward from the hips so that his near shoulder is firmly against her trunk. She can then lean across his back and grasp the outsides of his elbows with her fingers underneath them (**Fig. 32**). To prevent

Fig 32 *Elbow hold*

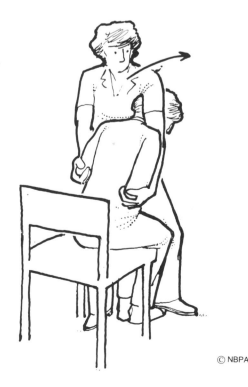

his trunk from rotating during the transfer, she locks his far shoulder by bringing her arm in front of it. This grip gives excellent control of the patient's movement. It should be perfectly comfortable, no pressures being exerted on his head or neck (Hollis 1991).

Handling-belt Hold

The nurse stands in front and to one side of the sitting patient, one foot beside him and the other in front, blocking the patient's knees and more particularly a weaker knee. Her thumbs can be inserted inside the waist-band of the patient's trousers or skirt and the garment then grasped with the whole hand. Alternatively, a wide, comfortable belt can be used round the patient's hips or waist and grasped by the nurse (**Fig. 33**), but it must be fastened tightly enough to ensure that it does not slip up round the chest. The patient

can support himself by pushing up on the arms of the chair or by putting his hands on the nurse's hips or assist by grasping the nurse's own belt.

Axillary Hold

The nurse stands facing the patient, with one foot beside the patient and the other in front, her knee 'blocking' the patient's knee. On the side near the nurse, she puts her hand over the patient's shoulder blade or, as an alternative she can insert her fingers from the back of the axilla. On the side away from the nurse she inserts her fingers as far as possible round the patient's chest under the axilla (**Fig. 34**).

For the last three holds it is essential that the patient is sitting well towards the front of the chair, leaning forward with his feet tucked in close to the chair, which will bring his centre of gravity over his feet.

Holds for Two Nurses

It should be remembered that when two people share a load, each of them is in effect supporting two-thirds of that load. In some situations the weight will be unevenly distributed, as for example in the Through-arm Lift (see Figure 60) when the nurse supporting the patient's trunk and shoulders will be more at risk than the nurse supporting the feet. These factors should be taken into consideration in the Assessment (Health and Safety Commission 1991).

Fig 33 *Waist hold using a handling belt*

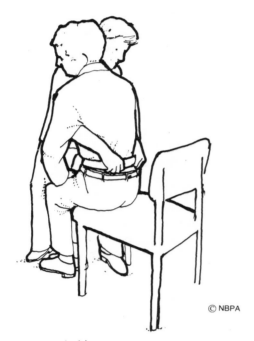

© NBPA

Fig 34 *Axillary hold*

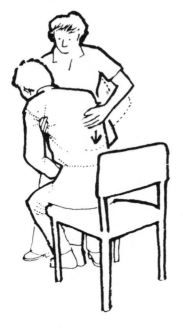

© NBPA

Fig 35 *Patient-handling sling*

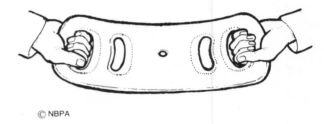

© NBPA

Fig 36 *Double wrist hold*

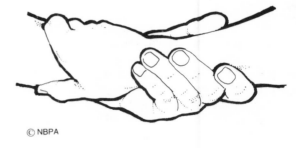

© NBPA

Fig 37 *Finger hold*

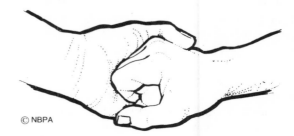

© NBPA

If nurses have to lift the whole weight of a patient manually, at least two nurses are required and they must have a secure grasp under the patient. A Patient-handling Sling (**Fig. 35**) should be used for this, in order to extend their reach and reduce the stooping action. In the absence of a Handling Sling, a Double Wrist Hold (**Fig. 36**) or a Finger Hold (**Fig. 37**) should be used.

Through-arm Hold

This is useful for controlling and supporting a dependent patient's trunk and shoulders, and can be used in different ways:

* By two nurses, one on each side of the patient. The patient should hold his forearms close to his body and in the case of any weakness, grasp his weaker wrist with the stronger hand. Facing in the same direction as the patient, each nurse puts her inner hand through between the patient's chest and arms from behind, and grasps the patient's forearm as near the elbow as possible, using the whole palm of her hand, not just the fingers (see Figure 52).

* By one nurse. The nurse then positions herself directly behind the patient and puts both her hands through to support his forearms (**Fig. 38**).

Holding the Walking Patient

Nurses are often expected to assist the patient when he starts to walk after a period of bed rest, after injury or following a stroke. The nurse should make a careful assessment, together with the physiotherapist, to determine exactly what the patient is able to accomplish either alone, when a walking aid such as a stick, crutches or a frame may be indicated, or with the help of one or more assistants. The results of this assessment must be passed on to the other nurses by means of a colour coding system or entry in the Care Plan.

The unsteady patient should wear a belt. The nurse, or nurses, should stand close to the patient on the weaker side, using the Palm-to-Palm Thumb Grip (**Fig. 39a**). On the right side of the patient the nurse holds the patient's right hand in her right hand and on the left, viceversa. The patient's arms should be straight, pressing down with his palm onto the nurse's palm with their thumbs interlocked (with a clinging patient the nurse may prefer to avoid the thumb hold – **Fig. 39b**). The nurse's other hand can be used to keep the patient's elbow straight, but without gripping his arm painfully or putting pressure under his armpit, or she can hold him round the waist. The nurse must be close to the patient to avoid unnecessary stress on her back, but also to support the patient, and both must face in the direction in which they are walking. She is then in a position to take the patient's weight through her hip rather than through her back, should he start to sag. If the patient feels unsteady the nurse maintains the Palm-to-Palm Thumb Grip, holds the

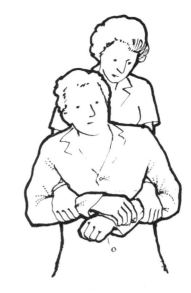
© NBPA

Fig 39a *Palm-to-palm thumb grip*

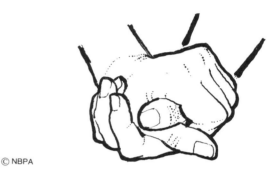
© NBPA

Fig 39b *Avoiding the thumb grip*

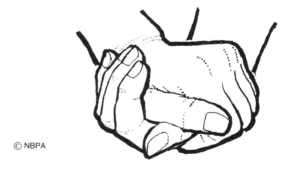
© NBPA

patient close with her other arm round his waist on his belt and blocks his knees with her leading leg; in this position the patient can be kept from falling with minimal effort (**Fig. 40**).

It is not uncommon for injuries to occur when unsteady patients are being escorted. The nurse must position herself in such a way that she can cope with him safely if he starts to fall. Again it is strongly recommended that the patient wears a belt to afford the nurse a secure hold should he start to sway. This

Fig 40 *Holding the walking patient*

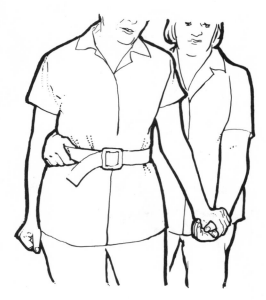

© NBPA

will also be of help for tall nurses escorting small patients.

If the patient is able to hold a walking frame but is weak, so that the nurse is unsure how far he can go, she can give the patient confidence simply by walking behind, pushing a chair which allows the patient to sit down immediately, should he have to stop. Similarly, a frail patient is likely to be more steady and confident if he has his walking practice on the return journey from the toilet, rather than on the way there, when he is trying to control a full bladder.

WARNING

The practice of the nurse pushing the patient's foot forward with her own foot or placing her foot under the patient's foot is dangerous. If the patient needs such assistance he is not yet ready for walking practice.

Chapter 12
The Bed

TYPES OF BED

Introduction

Back strain is frequently incurred due to inadequate space round the bed. Nurses should not have to move heavy furniture in order to obtain access to the patient without reaching. Bedside lockers should move easily away from the bedside on freely moving wheels so that helpers can get alongside the patient when lifting. Dependent patients should never be nursed in beds which are against the wall. In hospital the 2.5 m bed centre recommendation (Department of Health 1986) should be adhered to as far as possible, and planned for when new wards are commissioned: "the minimum dimension of each bed space should be 2.5 m by 2.9 m (long axis of bed) and there should be no intrusion into this space". Those responsible for the registration of nursing homes should draw up similar guidelines to ensure adequate space for safe handling. Brakes, wheels and height-adjustment mechanisms must be properly maintained and an efficient system for repair established so that no faulty bed is left in use. The design of backrests and brakes should allow ease of use and all moveable parts of the bed should move freely and smoothly. In particular, easy access to brakes should be ensured. Beds must be compatible with the hoists used in the ward or bedroom.

Where divan type beds are used in order to maintain a normal environment, they must be of adjustable height if the patient or resident cannot move himself. Duvets should be used on low beds to reduce the amount of stooping for the bed makers.

In the home, advice should be given to the carers on a safe nursing environment both for their own and the nurses benefit. Patients are often nursed at home on low double beds against the wall possibly with a cluttered bedside table jammed against the bed. This scenario makes the nursing of highly dependent patients extremely hazardous. A tactful request for a more suitable bed in more spacious surroundings may have to be made, or an order put in to the loans department for a hospital type bed, or an electrically operated home care bed. As with the installation of hoisting equipment, if the patient's family will not

agree to improve the environment, the care manager should intervene on behalf of her staff, and the consultation procedure to be followed in such an eventuality should be written into the local policy for patient-handling.

There is a large variety of beds available for nursing care. The nurse needs to be knowledgeable about the range and should know how to select a bed which is suitable for any particular patient. It is strongly recommended that local Equipment Monitoring Groups be set up to collect information and make recommendations about the purchase of beds and other equipment to budget holders.

Variable Height Beds for Hospital Use

Under no circumstances should patients today be nursed in fixed-height beds. The variable height type was originally designed by the Kings Fund in about 1966 and has since been manufactured by many different firms. These beds greatly reduce the strain of patient-handling. They range in height from 20″ to 32″ (50 cm to 80 cm), operated either electrically or mechanically, and have removable head and foot boards to facilitate patient-transfers. The nurse should, however, beware of the following disadvantages:

- The width of the bed (3 ft, 90 cm) requires the nurse to lean well forwards in order to reach the patient.

- Handle operated, variable height mechanisms cause the nurse to stoop with a twisted spine and, if the bed is occupied, the effort required in this dangerous position is considerable. Pedal operated beds should be selected when purchasing.

- Hydraulic jacks are notorious for breakdowns. Mechanical jacks with a guarantee should be selected.

- Back rests are often awkward to operate for the nurse who will be standing with her back twisted. Gas spring mechanisms which raise the top section of the bed frame are preferable.

- Braking systems can cause back strain either through failure when a patient is being moved or because the levers are difficult to reach or operate.
- 'Strippers' for the bed clothes frequently become jammed.
- The bed chassis may obstruct the positioning of a mobile hoist.

Local equipment policies should include a specification for purchase of beds in order to avoid as many of these pitfalls as possible.

Variable Posture Beds

These have a varying number of mattress platforms which enable the occupant to vary his own position in bed from lying to sitting, thus reducing the need for nurses to move patients. There are different types designed for hospital or domestic use. Some have adjustable head, leg and central hip sections; double or single size; remote electrical or manual adjustments.

Special Beds

In addition to the Kings Fund bed, there is a group of special beds designed for special purposes where patient-handling needs to be minimised, such as following severe injuries or prostration and where pressure sores occur which defy normal care. The main benefit is derived from the type of mattress the patient lies upon.

The Clinitron Bed

This bed is only available on hire. It is heavy and unusually large, and its height cannot be adjusted, but it has a built in platform for the shorter nurses to stand on. The mattress section consists of particles which are fluidised by warm air being pumped through them; when the pump is switched off the mattress solidifies. The following handling problems with this type of bed should be noted:

- **Getting the patient into or out of the bed.** This bed would normally be occupied by patients requiring continuous bed rest. A hoist should be used to get them into and out of it.
- **Moving the Patient.** Because of the flotation effect of the bed, it is unnecessary to move the patient up or down the bed. If the patient has moved too near to the bottom of the bed there is a special sliding sheet supplied with the bed which enables the nurses to pull the patient back without lifting.
- **Inserting a bed pan.** This is done by pushing part of the mattress away to make a space for the bed pan. The mattress can then

be solidified. Similarly, the patient can be rolled into a side lying position for dressings to be carried out.

- **Sitting the patient up.** A cushion which is provided can be pushed in behind the patient.

The Water Bed

In effect this is a tank full of warm water which is contained in a membrane. As with the Clinitron beds the patient does not have to be moved up or down and any movement which does have to be made such as rolling for washing, dressing etc., can be effected by displacing the membrane under the patient.

WARNING

The Clinitron and Water beds can cause back strain in nurses if they are treated like conventional beds. Any problems should be anticipated when ordering and it is essential that staff should be instructed in their use by the supplier when they are installed.

Pressure Relieving Mattresses

Water Mattresses are mattresses of varying types filled with water, some of which sit on top of the conventional mattress, and others which sit directly on the bed frame. They provide effective pressure relief but nurses should be aware that they are heavy to lift when the bed is being made, and ensure that they protect themselves by adjusting their posture when doing so.

Other pressure relieving mattresses include alternating air filled mattresses, cut foam mattresses, low air loss mattresses, and mattresses made of silicone padding. All these should be approached with care and forethought by the nurse when handling the patient. Although they have great advantages for the patient, they often obstruct the use of handling devices and sometimes prevent the nurse from putting her knee on the bed to get close to the patient.

Turning Beds

There are many of these on the market and they should always be provided when heavy and highly dependent patients are nursed. Types include electrically or manually operated turning frames. Turning frames with net mattresses and net suspension beds are extremely beneficial for nursing patients with major trauma, extensive burns and pressure sores.

Electrically operated turning and tilting beds are often supplied in Intensive Care Units; these beds are often particularly wide and nurses should be aware of the need to lean far over to reach the patient. Patient-handling slings and sliding sheets should be used to move the patient whenever possible. Care should also be taken in these units to organise equipment so that patient-handling is not obstructed.

Stand-up Beds

For patients who have fixed hip joints, then such items as the stand-up bed may be the answer to independence. The bed mattress and frame is electrically controlled so that it pivots on a central mechanism bringing the footboard flat on the floor and the bed to a vertical position. The patient can then shuffle on to the footboard, and from there onto the floor. He can then operate the controls so that the bed returns to its horizontal position. A bar will hold the bedding (usually a quilt) and pillows can be attached with tapes or Velcro to prevent them falling.

This stand-up bed is equally useful for some orthopaedic wards where patients undergo back surgery and whose post-operative management requires the avoidance of any flexion or movement of the spine.

Stryker Turning Bed

The Stryker Turning Bed was designed originally as an orthopaedic turning frame but is sometimes used in other fields. A second mattress is positioned on the frame, over the top of the patient; both mattresses are turned completely over with the patient sandwiched in between; the first mattress is then removed. By this means it is possible to turn the patient from a supine to a prone position and *vice versa*, with minimum disturbance to the patient and minimum effort for the nurse.

Devices to Prevent Patients Slipping Down in the Bed

The patient who constantly slips down in the bed makes heavy work for the nurse. As well as the variable posture beds mentioned above, there are other ways of preventing this from happening such as the use of polystyrene cushions. Nurses should also consider leaving him where he is, his pillows propped up by a portable back rest.

PROCEDURES FOR HANDLING ON THE BED

Equipment Required for Handling Patients in Bed

- variable height bed with foot pump mechanism is essential for ease of handling.
- a monkey pole, lifting blocks, and rope ladder to help the patient move himself.
- patient-handling slings, sliding devices to help the nurse move the patient.
- female urinal and Charnley wedge to remove the need to lift.
- overhead hoist for moving heavy patients in bed.

An overhead (ceiling or gantry) hoist is easier to use than a portable hoist, and it has been observed that nurses will use the former more readily. It is strongly recommended that tracking or gantries should be installed over at least two beds in all medical, surgical, orthopaedic and elderly care wards, and in any specialised areas where heavy dependent patients are likely to be nursed; and that where new wards and hospitals are commissioned, ceilings should be made strong enough to take tracking.

Sliding Devices for Moving the Recumbent Patient

There are many of these on the market now, and they should always be used in preference to a manual lift. The Easyslide and Handylet are rollers made of low friction padded material, the Lateral Transfer Board and the Patslide are thin flat boards, and the Patient Roll Board is a light weight roller. As with any other piece of equipment, they should be tried out before purchase, in order to obtain the type most suitable for the intended task.

Some sliding devices such as the Mini-Slide, a small version of the Easyslide, can be adapted to transfer the patient in a sitting position.

Turning the Patient

Whilst the patient should be encouraged to turn himself in bed (Chapter 8) it is often necessary to turn the patient for change of positions, for skin care, sheet changing and insertion of bed pan.

It is recommended that patients who need regular turning be nursed on one of a variety of turning beds, or by using an Easyslide (see Figure 24a) which can easily be used by relatives nursing a patient at home. A sheepskin or strong draw-sheet can also be used to turn the patient, and both should have a piece of polythene sheeting – which may be improvised with a strong plastic bag in the home – placed underneath to facilitate sliding.

Two patient-handling slings (see Figure 35) can be used where there is no sheepskin or draw-sheet. These are positioned under the patient's thighs and lower back. Feet, head and shoulders are moved first and then nurses on either side hold the slings to pull and roll the patient's pelvis and trunk.

Lifting is unnecessary; turning only involves rolling and sliding the patient. The rule is that the nurse rolls or slides the patient towards, never away from her. No nurse should every reach forward to move a patient away from herself.

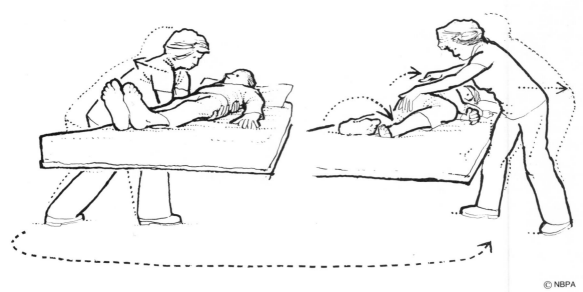

© NBPA

Fig 41 *Turning the patient with one nurse*

In most cases the patient will have to be rolled onto his back and then moved by use of the draw-sheet to the side of the bed, so that when turned he comes back to the centre of the bed. Use of the draw-sheet ensures that any friction occurs between the draw-sheet and the undersheet, not between the patient's skin and the undersheet. Movement to one side of the bed is done in three separate stages; moving first the head and shoulders, then the legs and lastly the trunk, which is most easily moved by means of the draw-sheet. In each case the nurse moves the patient towards herself, with her feet apart and one in front of the other for balance, and enabling her to use her body-weight. A second nurse may be required to ensure that the patient does not roll over the edge of the bed and may help position the feet, steady the head etc. With a heavy patient, two nurses may be needed to slide his trunk and hips – both pulling from the side – whilst a third nurse helps from the opposite side.

Then with the patient on the right side of the bed, he is rolled to lie in the centre on his left side; first preparing the head and shoulders to ensure that the left arm is not trapped; next his legs, crossing the right over the left and flexing the right hip; and then, using the knee and shoulders as levers, rolling the trunk.

If it is absolutely necessary for the nurse to insert her arms under the patient to move him to the side of the bed, she should push her hands palm downwards into the mattress to ease them through and then turn them upwards (**Fig. 41**). When rolling the patient towards her she should extend her arms further than

is necessary across the patient's trunk and then bring them back onto his body so that she can use her body-weight to move him.

Where there is a risk of the patient falling from the bed, a bed rail should be provided. These should not however, be used to prevent patients from getting out of bed. This rail can then be used to stop the patient rolling out if he is being turned single-handed. In the home, an item of furniture can be used. Always move the patient towards you, never away. Many patients need to be left in a semi-recumbent position, and in that case it is easiest to lift them with the appropriate method up the bed, but placing them nearer to one side of the bed than the other, and then roll them as described above.

Remember that side lying in this position can be uncomfortable because the trunk is flexed sideways, and the patient is therefore likely to try to roll onto his back. Frequent turning in a lower position is preferable, and indeed secretions at the base of the lungs will be drained more effectively as long as the patient's breathing is not embarrassed in this position (Hough 1984).

In cases where rolling presents a risk, for example following hip surgery, a Charnley abduction wedge can be used (see Figure 93) and the patient rolled safely. If necessary this procedure should be discussed with the surgeon in the light of the obvious risks to the nurses if they are required to lift manually for whatever reason; and an instruction entered into each individual Care Plan.

Insertion of a Bed Pan

If the patient cannot 'bridge' (see Figure 92) or raise his buttocks by holding onto the monkey pole (Fig. 42), a bed pan should be inserted by rolling the patient towards the lifter, positioning the bed pan and rolling him back onto it.

Fig 42 *Using a monkey pole to bridge*

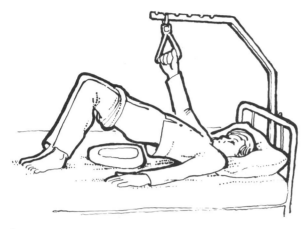

© NBPA

If for some reason this is not feasible and a heavy patient has to be lifted, then a hoist should be used. Alternatively, with a lightweight patient, two nurses, each with a knee on the bed, can use handling slings to raise his buttocks momentarily while a third nurse inserts the bed pan.

The nurse should remember that the patient feels extremely precarious when left sitting on a bed pan and she should ensure that he has either a cot-side or hand-blocks (see p.61) to hold onto.

Sitting the Patient Forward in Bed

Sitting the patient forward in bed for attention to pillows, back washing etc., a seemingly simple procedure, can cause injury, as the weak patient has a tendency to flop backwards against the nurse.

Whenever possible a 'rope ladder', or alternatively a rope with knots in it should be fixed to the bottom of the bed to allow the patient to pull himself forward.

With Two Nurses

One nurse faces the patient, places her nearest knee on the bed and clasps him round the trunk. She brings him forward by sitting back on her heel and is able to hold him comfortably against her while the second nurse sees to the pillows etc (Fig. 43).

With One Nurse

Facing the patient, she clasps him round the shoulder blades and eases him into a sitting position. She then moves her near arm across his back to keep him forward, placing her hand on the far side of the bed as a strut (Fig. 44). This leaves her other hand free to adjust the pillows.

Additionally, a draw sheet or an additional folded sheet can be placed beneath the lying patient from the shoulders down to their hips. The top edges of the sheet can then be used as a sling for the nurse to grasp and pull the patient towards her into a sitting position (Fig. 45).

Alternatively, for both of these two procedures the nurse familiar with the neuromuscular approach (see p.51 Chapter 9) will ease the patient forward from behind by applying hand pressure at the base of his shoulder blade and using her body-weight against his.

Fig 43 *Sitting the patient up in bed – with two nurses*

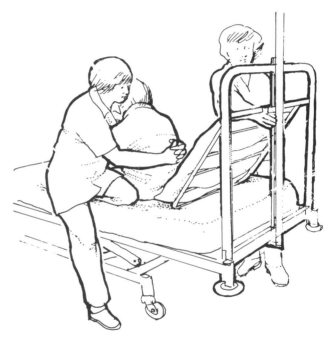

© NBPA

Fig 44 *Sitting the patient up in bed – with one nurse*

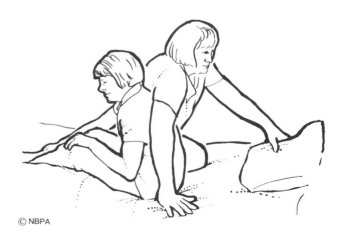

© NBPA

Fig 45 *Using a draw sheet to sit the patient up in bed*

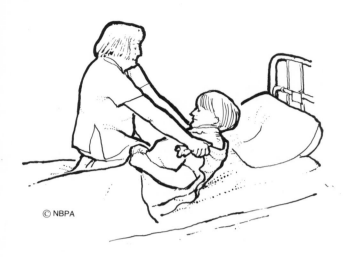

© NBPA

Fig 47 *Patient handblocks*

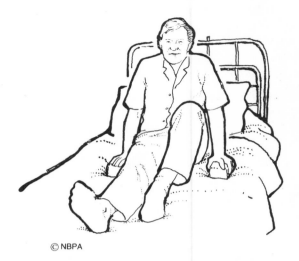

© NBPA

Fig 46 *Using a chair as a back rest*

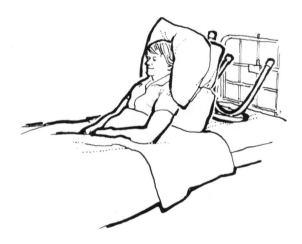

© NBPA

Moving the Patient up the Bed

The first question is, does he need to be moved, or could he be propped up where he is with extra pillows, with a portable back rest or with a small chair turned upside down to serve as a back rest? (**Fig. 46**). The second question is can he move himself up the bed? (For independent movement see Chapter 8).

Some patients, for example younger people with legs in plaster or traction, will be able to hold onto a monkey pole and push themselves up the bed by digging one or both heels into the bed.

Other patients will be able to use two hand-blocks (**Fig. 47**) to raise themselves clear of the bed and push back in the same way. In the home, hand-blocks can be easily improvised with two or three paper back books tied together with a long scarf or crepe bandage.

If the nurse is assisting the patient while he is using a monkey pole, care should be taken that he does not swing away from her, putting her in a position of

postural stress. Generally speaking, it should not be used where the patient is being lifted, as it causes the patient to reach upward and backward, instead of leaning forwards which makes lifting easier for the nurses. There is also a risk of the patient leaving go of the monkey pole or dropping his weight suddenly onto the nurses.

However, if there is a Balkan Beam attached to the bed for traction attachment, two nurses can lift a patient who is holding onto a monkey pole with minimal stress, if with their lower hands they hold onto a patient handling sling placed under his thighs and with their upper hands they hold onto the Balkan Beam to obtain leverage.

Hoists tend to be under used for this procedure, mainly because not enough ceiling hoists are provided. Where there is a ceiling or gantry hoist, the patient is moved up or down the bed simply by raising him up and moving the bed backwards or forwards as required, then letting him down again.

Similarly, sliding sheets should be put to much greater use than is the case at present. Sheets made of low friction material, with handles are available. The patient who is very ill or in pain when moved can be nursed on one of these so that he can be eased up the bed by the required number of nurses with his weight comfortably distributed.

As a temporary measure, a draw-sheet or sheepskin that the patient is lying on can be used to slide the patient up the bed.

Moving Patients up the Bed in their Own Homes

District nurses and home carers are greatly at risk when attempting to move patients up the bed on their own. The patient should be slid rather than lifted if possible. This may mean loosening the undersheet and pulling him up on that; or putting in a piece of polythene – a large plastic bag is useful – under a drawsheet. If the patient is capable of taking a little weight, it is better to help him put his legs over the side of the bed and then to move sideways up the bed and in again when he is near enough to the pillows.

Manual Lifts up the Bed – the Last Resort

Patients may have to be lifted manually. Handling slings should always be used; with the only exception of the Shoulder Lift when used for a patient of less than 112 lb (50 kg), when the nurse with average length arms may find that she actually reduces her leverage by using a sling. In most cases, one of the handler's knees should be placed on the bed to enable her to get closer to the patient.

The Two-Sling Lift

This is suitable for the patient who cannot sit forward. But he should be able to lift his head and, if not, a third nurse must hold his head gently forward to prevent it from being pushed into the pillows. One sling is placed at the patient's hip joints so that it supports the upper thighs. The second sling is placed at the upper waist so that it supports the rib cage. The slings enable the nurses to stand erect as they move the patient, provided the bed height is adjusted to halfway between hips and knees. Alternatively, the nurse may prefer to get closer to the patient by putting a knee on the bed (**Fig. 48**) in which case the bed can be lower.

Fig 48 *Two-sling lift*

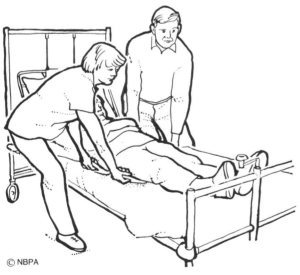

© NBPA

The same method can be improvised with the use of a draw-sheet (**Fig. 49**) instead of handling slings, as a temporary measure to make the patient comfortable. Alternatively a Lifting Sheet can be introduced.

With any manual lift up the bed there is a risk that the patient's heels will be dragged over the sheets. If a particular patient's heels are at risk or already showing signs of pressure, protection is required. Either he should be wearing sheepskin heel protectors, or a Mini-slide or a piece of plastic sheeting

placed under his heels will slide with them. It may be necessary to ask a third nurse to hold his feet.

Fig 49 *Improvising – using a draw sheet*

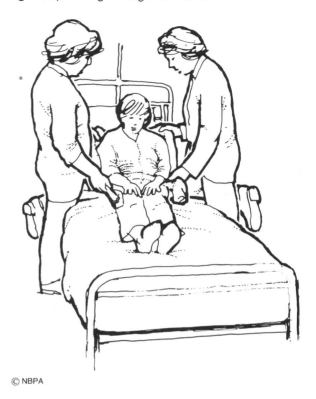

© NBPA

The Shoulder Lift*

This lift may be used for lifting a patient up a bed, when transferring from bed to chair or *vice versa*. It should not be used if the patient is too heavy to be lifted manually, if he cannot sit up, or if he is confused. It may not be suitable for those patients with injury, disease or pain in the shoulder, chest or upper back; nor should it be used post-operatively for patients who have had hip surgery. This lift enables nurses to hold the patient closely while using one arm as a strut and so reducing the stress in the spine. If possible, the bed should be adjusted to a level just above the knee and the brakes applied. The patient is assisted to a sitting position, and while one nurse supports him, the other can adjust the pillows, etc.

The nurses position themselves one each side of the bed facing the head of the bed, with the inside knee and foot on the bed, so that their knee is level with the patient's buttocks.

From behind the patient, the nurses press their near shoulders into the patient's chest wall under his axilla, while the patient rests his arms on their backs. The nurses' near arms are then passed under the patient's thighs as close to the buttocks as possible. Each nurse then firmly grips the other using a Wrist or Finger Grip (see Figures 36 & 37). Where there is difficulty in reaching the other nurse's hand or the nurse feels she is stretching her arm out awkwardly

---

* Formerly known as the Australian Lift

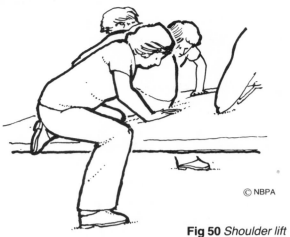

Fig 50 *Shoulder lift*

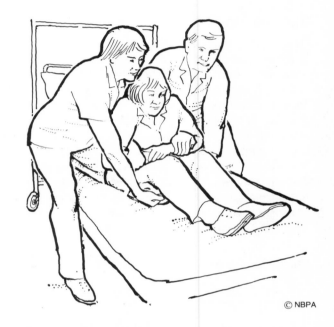

Fig 51 *Shoulder lift – both knees on bed*

behind her, then grasping a towel or a Patient-handling Sling beneath the patients thighs will ease the nurses' posture. The nurses' other hands are placed on the bed behind the patient to relieve stress on the nurses' trunks. The elbows are flexed ready to take the weight during the lift. Under no circumstances should the forward hand be placed on the patient's back or moved from its supporting position. The nurses should raise their heads as they lift to maintain the cervical curve and to point their bodies in the direction of the move (**Fig. 50**). Sometimes nurses prefer to obtain leverage by placing their free hands on the bed head, and this practice has been shown to cause no greater truncal stress (Scholey 1983) if the patient is already quite near to the pillows.

When the leading nurse gives the command to lift, the nurses kneel up straightening the elbows of their supporting arms to power the lift. Their standing legs act as both pivot and thrust for the lifting movement. The patient is lifted clear of the bed, and then lowered by bending the standing leg and supporting elbows. The patient should only be moved a short distance at a time, so that the patients hips are between the nurses propped arms on the bed.

If the patient is on a double bed one nurse will have to kneel with both knees on the bed (**Fig. 51**) and as her posture will be unstable she must take extra care by not attempting to lift too far, making sure that the outside knee is in advance of the inside knee.

The Through-arm Lift

This enables two nurses, one on either side, to 'parcel up' the patient more effectively by holding him forward in a sitting position with the Two-nurse Through-arm Hold (see page 71). They face the bottom of the bed and place the inside knee on the bed behind the patient. The inside hand goes through the space between the patient's chest and upper arm and grasps the patient's forearm near the elbow using a palmar hold. With their outside hands they grasp the handling sling placed under his thighs and lift the patient back towards them, sitting back on their heels as they do so (**Fig. 52**). The patient should not be lifted further than their knees since this would involve rotation of their spines.

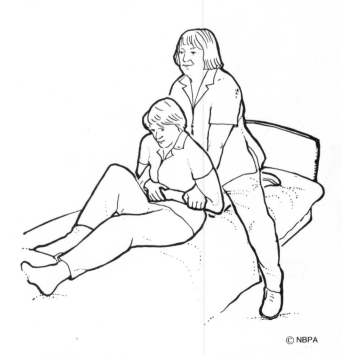

Fig 52 *Through-arm lift – two nurses*

Fig 53 *Through-arm lift – one nurse and patient helping.*

When a nurse is on her own, she may consider using the One nurse Through-arm Hold as described on page 71 (**Fig. 53**) However, unless the patient is exceptionally light and able to assist, the truncal stress will be very high. It is safer to assist the patient to sit on the edge of the bed and move himself sideways up the bed and then get in again.

The Combined Lift

This is a combination lift using a sling, for the patient who has one stiff or painful shoulder. Both nurses should place a knee on the bed, but they face in opposite directions. One nurse uses a Shoulder Lift and the other places her hand under the patient's sacrum as shown in **Figs. 54a & b**. The sling is placed under the thighs.

Non-weight Bearing Transfers to and from the Bed

Use of an Overhead Hoist

Patients who cannot take any of their own weight or use a sliding device to get in and out of bed should have the use of a hoist preferably of the overhead type (see Chapter 10).

At first, patients may be self-conscious and nervous about using a hoist; a tactful and sensitive approach is paramount when introducing it. Privacy and dignity must be maintained and the patient should understand that he can control events by asking the nurse to let him down, or to go more slowly at any time. The nurse must be absolutely confident in its use. If she fumbles or looks uncertain, the patient will be fearful and reject it.

Points to remember:

- check that the hoist is designed to take the patient's weight and is in working order.

- attach the sling so that as far as possible the patient is in a normal sitting position or the position most comfortable for his condition.

- avoid letting the patient swing like a pendulum by positioning the centre of the spreader bar close to the patient's centre of gravity.

- ensure that there is no uncomfortable pressure under the arms or thighs.

- ensure that the helpless patient's head is supported and protected and that his feet do not get knocked.

Transfers in the Absence of a Hoist.

Sliding Board for the Seated Patient

This is a smooth rectangular shape, normally of wood, which is bevelled at its narrower edges (**Fig. 55**).

Fig 54a *Combined lift for patient with stiff or painful shoulders – from the rear*

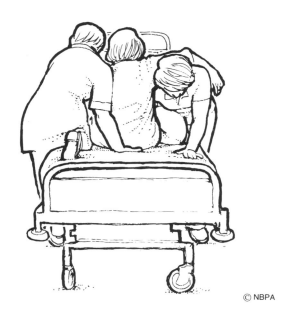

© NBPA

Fig 54b *Combined lift for patient with stiff or painful shoulders – from the front*

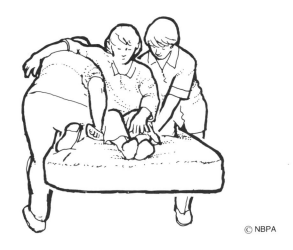

© NBPA

Fig 55 *Use of a sliding board transfer*

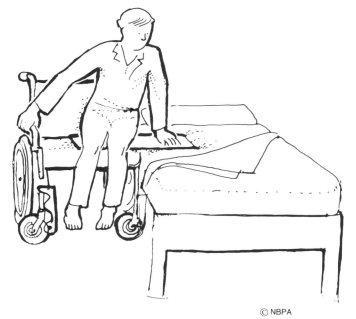

© NBPA

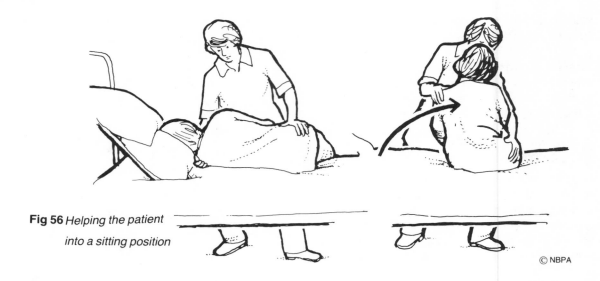

Fig 56 *Helping the patient into a sitting position*

© NBPA

The patient with good upper limbs can place the board beneath his hips as he sits in the wheelchair and across onto the bed or *vice versa*. He can then readily slide himself across to the adjacent surface. The furniture and surfaces for transfer must be of similar heights.

An angled sliding board is now available. This enables the user to move to an adjacent surface where there is a slight obstruction such as when getting in or out of a car which has rally type seats, or for some toilet transfers.

If the patient requires assistance for this transfer, it is best given by maintaining his trunk in a forward position, perhaps with the help of a transfer belt (see page 60).

The Shoulder Lift

This is suitable for a patient weighing up to eight stones, who can sit up. He should be helped to a sitting position and his legs swung round to hang over the side of the bed (**Fig. 56**). This is best achieved by asking him to roll, with help if necessary, towards the side from which he will be lifted. One nurse moves his feet over the edge and she can then pivot him into a sitting position by supporting him under his shoulder blade and applying hand pressure on his far hip. The two nurses join hands under his thighs near the buttocks (or use a handling sling), then position their shoulders under the patient's shoulders supporting the chest wall, his arms lying over their backs. Their supporting hands are placed on the bed behind the patient's buttocks with their elbows flexed (**Fig. 57a**). Then with their feet apart, on the word of command, they lift by straightening their knees and by pushing off with their supporting arms to come to a standing position. It is essential that they straighten up completely before moving any further. Their free hands can now support the patient's back as they carry the patient to the chair or commode (**Fig. 57b**). Timing is equally important for lowering the patient. For this the nurses must be ready, using their supporting hands on the arm or seat of the chair, and lower by bending their knees and supporting elbows. They should beware of putting their supporting hands on the top of the backrest of the chair when lowering, as the chair may tip (**Fig. 57c**).

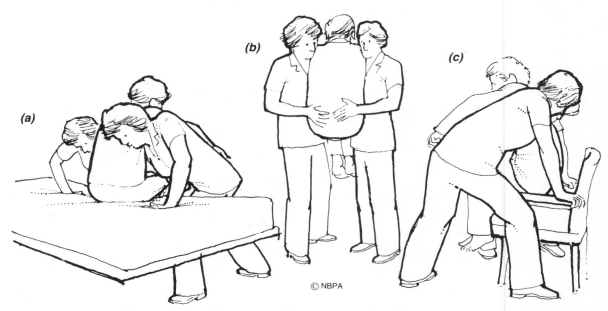

© NBPA

Fig 57a-c *Transferring the patient from bed to chair, chair to toilet and viceversa with two or more nurses*

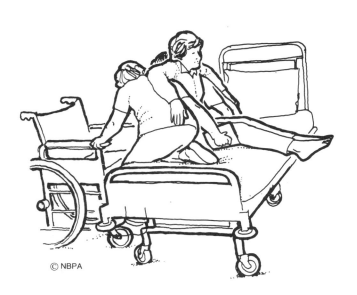

© NBPA

Fig 58 *Shoulder lift from bed to chair*

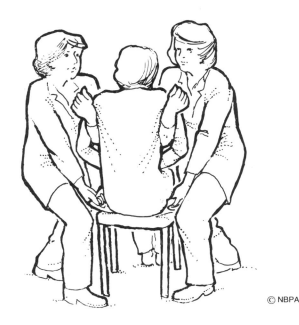

© NBPA

Fig 59 *Cross-arm lift*

When a patient has to be transferred to a high-backed wheelchair from a bed, the chair is brought with the front of it aligned with the side of the bed, and its wheels locked. The patient is then sat up with his back to the chair and his legs across the bed. The nurses then use a Shoulder Lift and lifting sling to move him back into the chair (**Fig. 58**).

The Cross-arm Lift

This is useful for the frightened, confused patient provided he is not too heavy for the nurses. They place a handling sling under his thighs as he sits on the edge of the bed, and position themselves in front of him, looking over his shoulders. **His weight is taken by the handling sling, NOT under his arms.** Their outside hands hold the sling, their inside arms support him under the axillae and he is thus moved round with control and security onto the chair (**Fig. 59**). Room must be left between the chair and the bed for the nurse to put her foot alongside the chair as she lowers the patient.

The Through-arm Lift

The Through-arm Lift is a useful alternative to the Shoulder-Lift, provided the transfer is not made to or from a chair with a high or obstructive backrest. When the transfer is made to a wheelchair, its back should be dropped down.

When two nurses are of unequal height, the taller nurse should take the head and shoulders because she will have a longer reach, and the shorter nurse the legs, because she will not have to stoop as far to lower them. Once the bed height is adjusted so that it is a little higher than the chair, the patient is moved to the side of the bed by means of the draw-sheet, ensuring that his head and shoulders are supported by one nurse's arm; his legs are left in the middle. The taller nurse then applies the Through-arm Hold

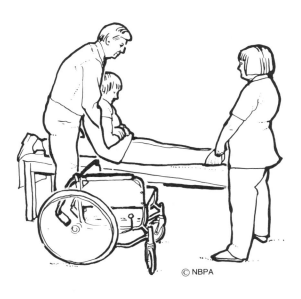

© NBPA

Fig 60 *Through-arm lift with two nurses of unequal height*

(**Fig. 60**) from behind him while he is at an angle to the side of the bed. The smaller nurse then places the chair conveniently close to the bed ensuring that there is not too big a gap, but not so close that the patient's elbow may be knocked on the side of the bed when lowered into the chair. The smaller nurse then stands facing the bed with feet one in front of the other and passes her hands under the patient's legs, ready to draw them towards her for the transfer. Alternatively she can lift in a more upright position by using a towel to lift the patient's legs. On the word of command, the legs are pulled over the side of the bed and the taller nurse lifts the patient's trunk from the side of the bed. The transfer is thus readily made, the nurses bending their knees to lower him into the chair.

Fig 61 *Using a Through-arm Hold and handling sling to transfer a patient who cannot stand, into a wheelchair.*

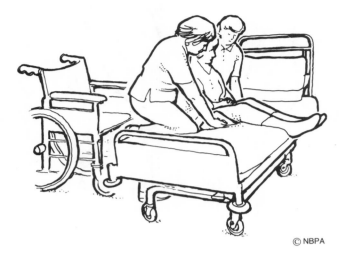

© NBPA

Another option is for two nurses to use a Through-arm Hold in combination with a patient-handling sling to move the patient into a chair turned towards the bed as in **Fig. 61**, which shows the first stage of the transfer, to the edge of the bed.

The Unconscious Patient

Handling the unconscious patient presents particular difficulties because he is inert, unable to co-operate in any way, and has little muscle tone. In effect, he is heavier than a conscious patient, because he slumps and sags when a conscious patient would not. Every part of him, and particularly his head, has to be controlled and supported.

The unconscious patient is at risk when being handled because he cannot shout out if it hurts and there is no reflex muscle 'guarding' of the joints, which can easily be dislocated. Long-term joint damage in the stroke patient very often starts when he is unconscious or semi-conscious, through careless handling.

The main principle, is to handle and lift the unconscious patient as little as possible, and avoid pulling about of any sort. For essential care, namely protection of pressure areas and moving the post-operative patient back to his bed, equipment should be used which distributes the patient's weight and minimises the need to lift.

The unconscious patient will need round the clock turning and so should be nursed on a turning bed. If one is not available he should be nursed on a lifting sheet or turning device such as the Easyslide (see page 56). Failing that a strong drawsheet or two patient-handling slings can be used, and the latter will facilitate moving him up or down the bed as well if necessary. Regular turning of a heavy unconscious

or semi-conscious patient without any form of equipment subjects nurses to cumulative strain and the risk of injury; it should not be expected of them. The risk is increased in Intensive Therapy Units where the beds are often wider than normal and the life support equipment inhibits free movement for the nurse.

In the operating theatre, routines for transferring patients should be carefully examined. Mechanised systems must be used to move the patient from trolley to the table. Until these are available a sliding device must be provided, both for the trolley/table transfer and the trolley/bed transfer, and all staff vigorously trained in its use.

The canvas and poles system is no longer recommended. It requires that the lift has to be made most often at waist-height. This makes great demands on the strength of the elbow flexors, and the knees can not be used to help with the lift. If canvas and poles are unavoidable, it is essential that the lifters can move their feet freely so that their backs do not have to be bent or twisted sideways while making the transfer. The poles must be long enough to ensure that the lifters do not have to stoop, as in the highly dangerous lift illustrated in **Fig. 62**. The spreader bars must be in place to prevent the canvas sagging; and headboards must be removed.

A canvas with one pole inserted can quite safely be used together with a sliding device for greater ease with a particularly heavy patient.

When a patient has to be turned face down onto the operating table, particularly onto a higher support, the risks are obvious. Ergonomically, it is deplorable and the system that requires it, is overdue for redesign. For example, the design of the operating table should allow for the posture of the patient to be adjusted after the transfer. Meanwhile at least three people are

Figure 62 *Dangerous use of canvas and poles*

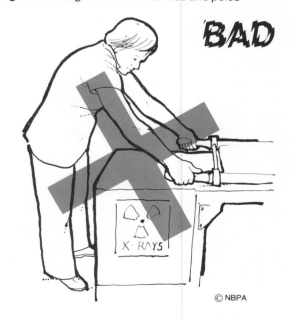

© NBPA

needed on each side of the operating table for such a transfer.

Special attention should be given for back care for staff working in operating theatres. Lifting of heavy weights under awkward conditions is one risk. Another is the requirement to hold a patient's limb, or maintain a difficult posture, for long periods. Both should be avoided if possible but time should always be allowed for recovery after exposure to these forms of postural stress.

Lifting dead bodies presents a hazard for the same reasons as does the unconscious patient. When transferring a body from the bed to the mortuary trolley, care should be taken to move obstructing furniture such as lockers. Alternatively the bed itself can be moved. A heavy body should not be lifted but should be slid across on a roller or on the undersheet. A particular problem with old trolleys is the fixed lid which obstructs access, and in this case purchase of ergonomically designed trolleys should be regarded as a priority.

TYPES OF CHAIR

Choice of Chair

The correct choice of an easy chair will contribute significantly to the independence of the user and will avoid the need for manual assistance from sitting to standing position. The basic design features of an easy chair should be viewed from an ergonomic approach to ensure that the design features are appropriate to the people who are to use it.

Chair Seat

The proper height of the seat depends on the leg length of the sitter and will range from 365-455mm (14½″ – 18″) (BS 4467 (1991)). As a guideline, the height should allow a person to place his feet comfortably on the floor. For a dependent patient, if a seat is too high the nurse will have difficulty in moving the patient back in the chair. For independent patients who can bring themselves forward in the chair without assistance, the height will increase their independence; and if the front edge of the seat is too high and is uncomfortable under the thighs, they can use a footstool. Placing cushions on the seat to raise the height is far from ideal as they make an unstable base and are liable to get uncomfortable. The inclination of the seat is important. If it is too level, it may allow the patient to slide forward too readily. The optimal inclination, combined with the softness of the seat, is to allow the patient to maintain his sitting posture without undue effort. The depth of the seat is a function of buttock-knee length in the range of 435-550mm (17½″ – 22″) (BS 4467 (1991)). If the seat is too long, the sitter will tend to slump, thus increasing the tendency to slide out.

The seat cushion is suspended on the chair frame by one of several methods. Too often the webbing or rubber strapping supporting the seat has sagged making the cushion soft. This will create difficulties for the person trying to rise to their feet. Choose a chair with a firm cushion or, if it is a favourite chair not to be discarded, then cut a piece of thick plywood the size of the chair frame to support the cushion on a firm base.

When choosing chairs for a communal sitting area, several different designs and widths of seat would assist a variety of users to chose for comfort. A seat that is too wide will allow people to fall or slump sideways into an unstable posture.

Chair Back

The chair back may be high to allow a user to support their head. A variety of neck and head cushions may make this more comfortable for the older user who has a forward stoop. High backed chairs will not allow people to be repositioned manually from behind the chair.

The chair back may have wings but these can sometimes encourage users to lean sideways and slump in a poor posture. Wings can also inhibit conversation when chairs are placed side by side.

Many users look for a chair back that has a lumbar cushion to support the lower spine. Others may prefer to use a loose cushion that can be placed exactly to provide comfort. This cushion may also help bring the person with a short leg length forwards in a deep seated chair.

The rake of the chair back may also influence comfort and independent use. The more inclined the chair back, the more difficult it is to rise. However, for those users with painful hip joints, a slight backward angle may give a more comfortable seated posture. If the chairback is too upright, the head tends to drop forward and the sitter then slumps.

Arm Rests

The arm rests of an easy chair should come well forward so that the users can grasp them to pull themselves into a position ready to stand. The front edge of the arm rest should be level with or in front of the seat-edge.

Padding on the top of the arm rests will allow elbow joints, which may be painful, to be supported and for some people to be able to shift their position in the chair by pushing down on their arms. Constant pressure from an unpadded armrest can induce a nerve palsy in the user's arm.

The height of the arm rests should allow the elbows to be supported and still allow the shoulders to be in natural alignment. Arm rests that are too high will elevate the shoulders and reduce the ability to use the person's arms to push down when rising. Too low and the user will slump sideways and depress the shoulder joint which may need supporting particularly following a stroke.

Chair Legs

There should always be at least 5" (130 mm) clearance beneath a chair. This will allow users to place their feet comfortably either when rising independently or for the helper assisting them. Should a hoist be used, then the chassis can pass beneath the chair frame to give a choice of positions in which to lift the user.

The front chair legs should be vertical and the rear legs should be angled backwards to increase the stability of the chair.

Should a chair need to be heightened then there are a number of methods available from a static or mobile raised base to individual sleeves into which each chair leg is placed. Blocks should be avoided since they are unstable when the patient knocks against a chair or sits down suddenly.

Reclining Chairs

This type of design of chair has become increasingly used as both an easy chair and a day bed. There are many types of reclining chairs available and care must be taken to select one which suits the needs of the user.

Reclined Position

Some recliners will allow the legs and feet to be placed in a position that will assist with oedema drainage (that is with the feet higher than the hip joints). But beware of the leg support that is too short and allows the feet to hang over the edge, causing skin pressure in vulnerable areas.

Chair Legs

Many recliners have castors to make them mobile but do not have chair legs. It should be assumed that this type of chair will often be used by the more dependent person and therefore the use of a hoist must be considered. Either a chair is chosen that the existing hoist chassis will go around from the front or side or a recliner with legs of 5" (130 mm) is used.

Supportive Chairs

There is a wide range of chairs available that offer a variety of special supportive seating positions. Some of these will have a tilting seat, be on a mobile base, have adjustable footplates and arms and trays for activities and feeding. Care should be taken when using this type of chair that it is not used to restrain the patient and that the patient is not left in an abnormal recumbent posture for long periods. When seeking advice about the choice and use of such chairs, care must always be taken to consider the method by which the user will get in and out of the chair. Many of these chair users will require the use of a hoist so that ground clearance may be a key design feature.

Riser Chairs

The range of chairs that have seats which rise and fall are widely used by people who have arthritic, painful or stiff joints. However they are unsuitable for those who do not have postural control of their heads or trunks. The basic designs fall into four categories:

- **the seat tilts upwards from the front.** These are often mechanically operated and may or may not have braking systems. The front edge of the seat height does not alter but the seat cushion rises up behind the user. Most of these designs require the chair mechanical systems to be chosen to fit the weight of the user. A person who is too heavy may not be able to operate the chair and a lighter person may find it unsafe. These chairs require the user to push on their arms to initiate the forward movement so those users with painful or weak arms will find this difficult. These chairs are therefore not always suitable for a group use environment.

- **the seat rises both upwards and forwards at an angle.** These are often the electrically powered types. At the press of one or two buttons the seat height is raised and the angle tipped forwards. These are useful where several people of different weights may be using them. They do not require the users to have strength in their arms.

- **the seat together with the back rises both upwards and forwards.** This design of chair is particularly suitable for those users who may have difficulty in their knee joints and placing their feet in the right position against the chair frame. Some users require support at their backs which rises with them while they are being placed up on their feet.

- **for users who cannot sit comfortably in any chair** because of their lack of flexion in arms, legs and spine, then there are chairs which will take a person from a standing to a reclining position in order for them to rest without having to be manually or mechanically assisted or lifted.

Chair Upholstery

While there is a wide choice of material coverings for chairs, many purchasers who are buying for group or multiple issue purposes will chose those fabrics which are water and stain resistant and easy to clean for reissue. Some users may find the vinyl type of materials assist them to slide and move themselves into positions of comfort or to rise but others will find that sitting for any period of time on such fabrics is sticky and uncomfortable.

PROCEDURES FOR HANDLING WITH CHAIRS

Rising from Sitting to Standing Independently

If a chair has been chosen to fit the patient, then this process of moving from sitting into the standing position will be considerably easier and often gives full independence to the patient.

The patient will lean forward with his head towards, if not over, his feet. He will then shuffle his hips from the back of the seat towards the front. His feet should be tucked under him with one foot placed slightly ahead of the other. The patient is able to push up on the arms of the chair to help him straighten his knees. As he comes up on to his feet, his head is raised up so that he stands erect. It is best to pause for a moment to check balance and to get a firm hold of his stick or walking frame (if used) before moving off.

All that is required of a nurse is to offer a reassuring presence and a verbal reminder of how to place head, hips, feet and arms.

Assisting a Person to Rise from Sitting

The nurse can either stand at the side of the chair (usually on the person's weakest side) or at the front of the chair to assist the person to move forward.

From the Front of the Chair

To assist the patient to ease his hips forward on the chair, the nurse bends her knees and hips to bring them in line with the chair seat if possible. The nurse's knees are either side of the patient's knees and her feet are slightly one in front of the other. This gives a wide stable base and allows the weight to move from the front leg onto the back leg as the person rises. The hips of the patient can be moved forward on the seat by gently rolling him from side to side. As one buttock is slightly raised off the seat so the nurse's hand under his thigh pulls it forward on that side. The rock to the other side then allows the

other leg to be pulled forward. Thus the hips are moved towards the front of the seat. The patient's feet are then placed under the leading edge of the chair seat ready to take weight. The nurse's arms are forward either grasping a belt at waist level or she uses the 'Axillary Hold' (see Figure 34). The patient's arms and hands are placed on his thighs or on the arms of the chair and he is asked to push down as the lift begins (Fig. 63). If he has a short term memory loss, is unable to follow instructions or **to prevent the habit of dragging on the lifters neck and shoulders**, then he can be given something to hold (a tissue or a soft object) so that his attention is caught and his hands do not interfere with the assistant. The nurse then gently starts to assist the patient to rock forwards and backwards until his weight is taken through his feet and he can stand.

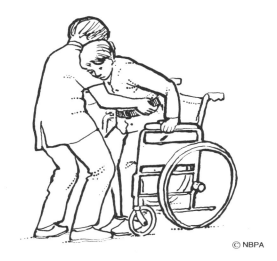

© NBPA

Fig 63 *Assisting a patient to stand using a belt*

From the Side of the Chair

A belt around the seated patient will enable the nurse to get hold of him without causing discomfort to shoulder or arm joints. If necessary the nurse helps him to shift his hips from the back of the chair to the front preparatory to standing. His feet are checked and placed beneath the leading edge of the seat and his hands are placed grasping the front of the chair arms. The nurse stands at the side of the chair facing the same direction as the patient. Her feet are placed with the outside foot forward and the nearside foot placed behind, level with the centre of the chair seat (or just behind the patient's hips). The nurse's nearside arm goes down and around his waist so that she can grasp a belt comfortably with her knees bent to prevent too much of a stoop. Her outside hand is brought across to support his arm. With both of them keeping their heads up and in the direction of the move, one or two gentle rocks forward should assist the person to stand.

Both of these assisted moves are easy if the chair is of a suitable height. Too low a seat increases the difficulty of the lift. The patient should not be left until he is comfortably seated, securely in the back of the chair.

Moving the Patient Back in the Chair

Patients with conditions affecting the locomotor system frequently slide down in their chairs. It is not usually necessary to lift them back up provided they are positioned correctly. The patient's knees must be flexed and his feet flat on the floor close to the chair, or on the step of a mobile chair. Hand pressure on the base of his neck will bring his trunk forward. He may then be able to move himself back by pushing his hand down on the arms of the chair and pressing down on his feet. If not, the nurse holds him in the sitting forward position preferably using a transfer belt or handling sling and uses her knees pressing on his knees to ease his pelvis to the back of the chair. She should keep her own knees and hips flexed throughout (**Fig. 64**).

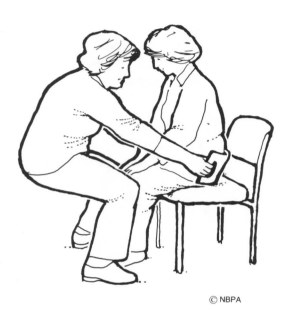

© NBPA

Fig 64 Moving the patient back in the chair

Relatives looking after a disabled patient at home should be encouraged to buy a 2″ wide leather belt to be worn around the patient's waist when he is being moved or helped to walk, so that they can hold him securely without pulling on vulnerable joints. It is possible to buy clothing which has a belt incorporated.

Transfer belts are not suitable on bare skin and are inadvisable in some patients with abdominal conditions or when pregnant.

Transfers for Partially Weight Bearing Patients with Two Nurses

Many frail unsteady patients need two nurses to support them when they are moving between two seated positions such as the bed, chair, or commode.

But first, nurses should check that the patient is indeed capable of taking some of his weight; if he cannot do so then, with most adult patients their body-weight will indicate that a hoist may be a more appropriate method to use.

The principles are as for assisting from the side of the chair described above. The chair is positioned so that the two nurses will have room to move but the distance between the two transfer surfaces should not be so great that the patient has to walk. The nurses both face in the same direction as the patient, close in beside the chair, with their nearside hands grasping the far side of the waist or lifting belt, or on the patient's furthest hip, crossing over the arm of their handling partner (**Fig. 65a**). Alternatively a Through-arm Hold can be used (see page 71). Their

Fig 65a&b Two nurses assisting a patient to stand

(a)

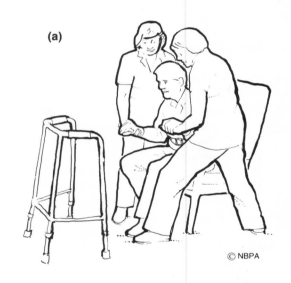

© NBPA

(b)

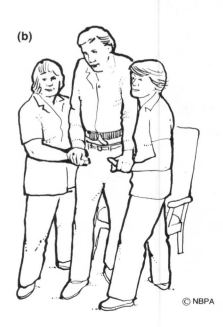

© NBPA

outer hands may either support the forearm of the patient, or hold the belt, leaving the patient free to push up with his hands on the arm of the chair. The nurses' feet are positioned so that their nearside legs are placed level with the patient's bottom on the chair, and their outer legs are braced forwards, just in front of the patient's feet on the floor. Both of the nurses' legs are slightly bent in order to allow themselves to place their arms around the patient's waist and to use their legs as a lifting force as they assist the patient to rise. The patient's feet are placed slightly apart and with one foot slightly in front of the other, so that he too will be balanced as he comes into an upright posture.

As the patient pushes himself up into a standing position, the nurses straighten their knees (**Fig. 65b**) and if necessary put pressure on his sacrum with their nearside hands to encourage him to straighten up. They then move round with the patient towards the waiting chair, commode or bed. For the patient who has one side substantially weaker than the other, the turning manoeuvre should be towards the weakest side. The nurses' feet are positioned ready to block either of his knees should they buckle and their hands ready to offer him additional support at the waist should he start to sway. If he actually starts to fall, they are in a position to let him gently down to the floor, keeping their own backs reasonably erect (see Management of the Fallen Patient Chapter 16).

When he reaches the chair and has his back to it so that he can feel the front edge of the chair against the backs of his legs, he should be encouraged to feel backwards for the armrests with his hands, to grasp them and then to lower himself as far back in the chair as possible. As he goes down, the nurses again relax their knees. It may then be necessary to help him to push his bottom further back into the chair. This is best done by rocking him from side to side while also gently easing his hips backwards on the seat.

WARNING

Pulling the patient into a standing position from the front, with the nurse's arms hooked under the patient's arms is DANGEROUS because of the pressure which this working posture puts upon the nurse's back. It is also likely to provoke resistance from the patient because of the discomfort caused to his shoulder joint.

Rocking

For patients who can co-operate and control their head and arm position, the stress of lifting can be eased by gently rocking them while seated as a preliminary to the move, whether to stand up or be transferred to another seat. Rocking gives the patient kinetic energy and by controlling this energy, the nurse is relieved of much of the lifting effort. The patient is assisted to the front of the seat by rocking him from side to side and pulling alternate legs forward. Then, with the patient's knees at 90° and his feet and knees together, the nurse stands with one foot beside him and the other foot in front blocking his knees. She then adopts one of the holds depending on the transfer to be made and on the patient's condition (see below). Now the patient is ready to be:

- assisted to a standing position

- moved through 90° from chair to wheelchair etc.

- or swung through 180° from a wheelchair to a toilet.

For each person the rocking follows the same principle. The nurse begins the movement by rhythmically swaying her weight backwards and forwards and thus, by virtue of holding the patient closely, sets him rocking backwards and forwards. There is no need to lift; simply by using her body-weight enough kinetic energy is transmitted to the patient to achieve the transfer. A few preliminary rocks are needed to set the rhythm, then with an increase in the movement, and the command: "READY, STEADY, UP", the transfer is made. If he is to stand up the nurse should brake his momentum once his weight is over his feet by exerting firm pressure on his sacrum. This will also cause him to straighten up.

Fig 66a&b *Rocking transfer for two nurses*

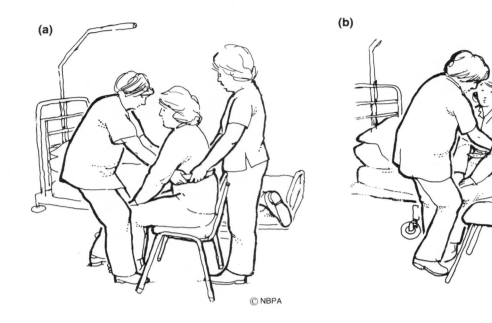

(a)

(b)

© NBPA

© NBPA

Rocking Transfer for Two Nurses

A rocking lift with the help of a transfer belt (or ordinary belt, at least 2″ wide, with a buckle or fastening) can often be used for a heavy and immobile patient with minimal assistance from a second nurse. To begin with the patient's feet are half turned in the direction of transfer. The second nurse stands behind the patient, with one knee on the bed if the patient is moving to or from a bed (**Fig. 66a**). As the first nurse rocks and swings the patient towards her, the second nurse eases the patient's buttocks round onto the chair or toilet (**Fig. 66b**). This is useful in a confined space because the nurses remain on the spot and only the patient moves.

The Rocking Pivot Transfer with One Nurse

Here the nurse is relieved of the patient's weight by using his feet as a pivot and his knees as a fulcrum. Both his feet and knees must be partially or totally blocked by her own feet and knees in order to achieve this (**Fig. 67**). These transfers are also used as a part of the rehabilitation process. In preparation it is important to match up bed/chair/commode heights and to ensure that the patient is sitting well towards the front of the chair or edge of the bed, leaning forward with his feet tucked in, i.e. 'nose over toes', which will bring his centre of gravity over his feet. The main principle of these transfers is to counterbalance the patient's bodyweight with the nurse's bodyweight. The nurse must therefore estimate beforehand whether her bodyweight is sufficient to do this.

The holds for use in the Rocking Pivot Transfers are the Elbow Hold, the Axillary Hold and the Belt or Waistband Hold (see Figures 33, 34). For patients with painful knees or ankles, a turntable may be used (see Figure 31).

Fig 67 *Rocking pivot transfer with one nurse*

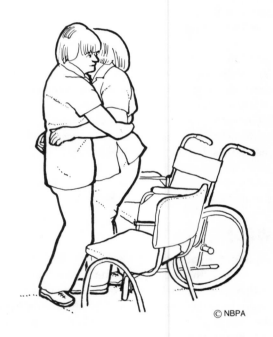

© NBPA

Assessment

The constraints imposed by both the environment and the personal nature of the activity, render toiletting a complex task and one that requires a careful assessment.

The Task

The basic task is for a person to be able to pass waste body products in the right place at the right time and with dignity and privacy wherever possible.

It is important to know how often the person wishes to use the toilet both for the passing of urine and bowel motions. In addition the control of women's menstrual flow can be considered since the changing of pads or appliances will involve a similar approach. Nurses should be aware of a safe emergency response to an urgent need as well as knowing how a person might normally be assisted. If someone suddenly becomes totally dependent, then a safe method of keeping the person clean, dry and yet relieved must be considered. An example of this may be a new patient referred to a Community Nursing Service who is found to be excessively heavy, non-mobile and unable to assist with any transfers. Until a full assessment can take place (for instance to provide a hoist and sling) then the response may have to be that the patient is catheterised until the correct handling equipment can be provided in order to effect safe transfers on and off the commode or WC.

The prescription and supply of the continence appliances should be checked as outdated or outgrown appliances often cause difficulties.

The Patient

Apart from knowing about the pattern and timing of the patient's use of the WC, information is needed about his general mobility and postural control.

In establishing methods of toiletting, the patient's wishes must be respected since this is the task,

above all others, that most people wish to do themselves and for which they are reluctant to seek assistance.

The patient needs to be aware of the different options open to him so that as the assessment takes place, he can contribute to the decision and to the Care Plan for toiletting.

The Environment

Toilet cubicles can be danger areas in many hospitals and residential and day care establishments. It is the site where many care staff are injured. Toilet cubicles have generally been designed and equipped without the benefit of either ergonomics or practical caring experience.

Commissioning officers should be aware that the standard door set width (30", 750 mm) is too narrow for an occupant-controlled wheelchair and for many of the push chairs. Without special consideration as to space and design, many staff will be struggling to move heavy and unsteady patients round through 180° turns in awkward and twisting positions.

Where the toilet cubicle does not allow for safe transfers, then the use of a mobile sanichair is a safer alternative. These types of mobile chairs can be used with a pan beside the bed (or in a private space) or can be pushed over the WC once the transfer has taken place in a more suitable, spacious environment.

Where commodes are used, they should be sited in a private area and placed in a position to aid a transfer. Too often a commode is used in a bedroom at night but the commode is not placed adjacent to the bed so that an elderly person wishing to use the commode has to struggle to reach it: a frequent cause of falls.

The Lifter

Carers helping with toilet transfers must be trained in the various options and techniques. They must be competent since this is when the patient is most vulnerable. Any equipment which is available must be safe to use with clear instructions.

Design of the WC

Some examples as to the sizes and designs for WC cubicles are laid out here. (Fig. 68a, b & c).

Where the dependency of the users has changed so that people now require more space, consideration must be given to the possibility of making two cubicles into one larger sized WC.

The height of a WC pan must enable an elderly or disabled person to place his feet on the floor while sitting. It is better to have a lower fixed-height and then to have alternative ways of raising the seat, than to have a fixed high seat which some people find too high and that a sani-chair will not push over. A raised WC seat can be supplied and these are available in 2″, 4″ or 6″ heights so that a seat to fit most people's needs can be found. This seat can either stay on the WC bowl or can be placed on the bowl when required. An alternative to the raised WC Seat is to replace the existing one with a fixed seat, fitted securely to the WC bowl. Both systems allow for personal cleansing. There is a wide choice of shape and design: horseshoe or front cutaway, oval or sloping sided. For the elderly, and disabled people who find that twisting to reach and clean themselves is painful and awkward, a range of bottom wipers is available. They extend the individual's reach and may be a useful solution to the problem of increasing dependence on others.

There are two basic methods of getting on and off the WC. Either from the side (a lateral transfer) or from the front (a frontal transfer). Space will need to be provided for these two options. In addition there may need to be a space behind the WC if the patient needs assistance for cleaning or clothing adjustment.

It may be possible for some people (particularly double, above knee, amputees) to do a forward transfer from their wheelchair on to the seat facing the cistern. Occasionally a backward transfer is possible but this requires a special back wheelchair canvas.

A cantilever (wall hung) WC allows easy access for transfer on and off the WC from a wheelchair since there is more floor space for both footplates and feet.

It is often preferable to have only a WC seat without a lid cover. Many people lean backwards while seated to gain support and it is not designed for it. Nor is it pleasant to lean against a soiled lid. Support rails with a back rest can be supplied and these are particularly useful where there is a high cistern with a down pipe at the rear of the WC. A high cistern is sometimes preferable to a low level suite since it will give an extra few inches of floor space.

Fig 68a *WC compartment for ambulant disabled people, door opening in*

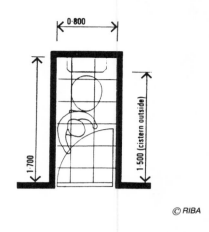

© RIBA

Fig 68b *Standard WC compartment for wheelchair users*

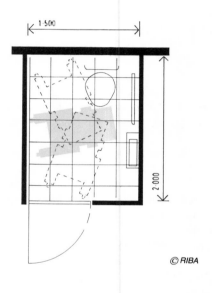

© RIBA

Fig 68c *WC compartment with freestanding WC*

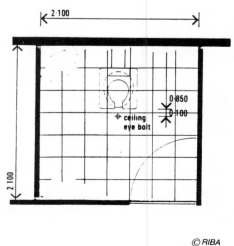

© RIBA

From "Designing for the Disabled" (Goldsmith 1976). Reproduced with the kind permission of RIBA Publications Ltd.

Fig 69 *Use of hand rails in toilet cubicle*

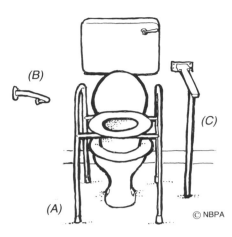

Rails to support the person using the WC can be provided in a number of ways (**Fig. 69**):

- a movable frame which may have a seat attached and may be adjustable in height **(A)**
- rails attached to the wall and floor and are fixed in position **(B)**
- rails that are fixed to the back wall and which are hinged so that they can be swung up towards the back wall thus creating more space when needed but swung down into place when required for a transfer **(C)**
- a floor fixed frame which can also be adjustable in height

The more adjustable and flexible the system chosen then the more people who will find the rail system useful. When considering the needs of users, some men may prefer to stand facing the WC and therefore they may require an upright rail close to one side. Others will sit on the WC and require rails that are best placed on the wall and which run from a point level with the centre of the WC bowl to at least 10″ (250 mm) forward from the edge of the seat.

Fixed toilet rails are suitable only where the toilet can be reserved for ambulant patients. They preclude transfers from wheelchairs and obstruct the handlers.

Cleansing

Cleansing after using the toilet can be achieved in a number of ways:

- by the use of paper. Folded interlocking paper sheets are easier to use by the one handed patient or the assistant. The container must be sited to the front of the person and not on the back wall behind them. Some WC support rails have an additional holder which will take a roll of paper so that it is within easy reach.

- a portable bidet is a plastic moulded dish which is designed to sit on top of the WC bowl. A small plastic jug can then be used to fill it with warm water. The person can then sit on it and wash themselves without struggling to keep on their feet. The used water can then be tipped down the pan.

- automatic WCs are available that incorporate a washing drying facility. A douche can be operated once the person is ready to be cleaned. This douche is of thermostatically heated water and is followed by a warm air dryer. While this type of cleaning system is welcome and practicable for most patients, those who suffer from muscular extensor spasm, particularly in the lower limbs, may find it unsuitable. However, the use of this type of WC reduces handling stress for nurses.

Commodes

There are many designs of commodes and as yet there is no British Standard set for their construction or required design features. There are five particular points that need consideration (**Fig. 70**):

Fig 70 *An ideal commode*

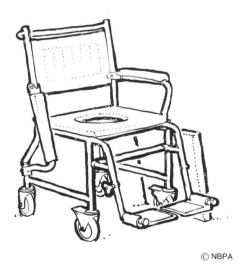

Legs

Legs should be splayed at the back to give stability to the chair but vertical in front to aid foot positioning. The commode may have adjustable height legs to suit individual users. The legs may have either non-slip feet or four castors, each with a brake. The castors will make it easier for assistants to move the commode around and it may also allow the commode to be used over a WC once the pan has been removed.

Pan

The Pan should be easily removable either from the top or from the seat. Some users prefer to be able to continue sitting and for the pan to be removed from underneath them via the rear of the seat. The top removal design may prevent a stoop or awkward posture by the assistant.

Seat

The Seat can be one of several designs:

- horseshoe shaped which sometimes makes self-cleaning easier
- conventional oval WC seat
- a round WC seat to fit the round pot
- a flat solid seat in which an oval hole has been cut. This is more suitable for the heavier seated person.

The seat must be wide and deep enough for the average seated adult while additionally wide and sturdy seats may be needed for the more obese patient.

Arms

The arms of the commode should be removable or hinged so that sideways transfers, e.g. on and off the bed, are easily achieved. However, they should not be so loosely fitted that a disturbed patient can remove them. Fixed arms get in the way of most assisted transfers and must be avoided. Some commodes which fasten to the bed frame are available (Fig. 71), and these give much stability to an independent transfer, particularly at night when there is minimal assistance available and the patient may be only partially weight bearing.

Fig 71 *Commode fixed to bed frame*

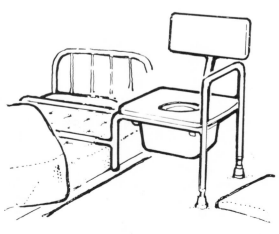

© NBPA

Back

The back may be padded and have handles to assist the handler in moving it around.

Multi-use

The choice of construction material may also enable a commode to be waterproof and therefore used as a shower chair. The patient can be transferred from bed on to the commode, wheeled over the WC or use the commode pan, and then showered while still sitting in the same chair. An example of this is the mobile sanichair supplied by several hoist manufacturers which also attaches to a lifting mechanism. An additional bed pan attachment converts these units into commodes.

Many commodes are chosen because they stack and take up little space when not in use. Commodes are most used at night and are removed from the bedside in the day time. Some are chosen as items of bedside furniture that look like conventional chairs. The practice of lifting and carrying commodes from the patient's bedside is stressful and should be discontinued.

When purchasing new commodes it is valuable to have a range of designs and sizes so that all patients' needs can be met.

Wheelchair Design

When people are transferring from wheelchair to WC then certain design features should be considered.

Back

For the few people who prefer to transfer backwards on to the WC then a split back canvas can be supplied.

Arms

Arms should be easily removable so that clothing can be adjusted, hoist slings easily positioned, or sideways transfers achieved.

Foot Rests

Foot rests should swing away from the front of the wheelchair and also detach. In assisting a person to transfer, there must be space on the floor to allow him to stand and move his feet freely.

Cushions

It is possible to have a wheelchair seat cushion that has a cut-out at the front edge which will allow patients to use a hand-held urinal in place beneath them while seated. Adapted clothing is required for this to be used successfully but it allows patients to micturate while sitting and without transferring.

Clothing

The management of clothing while toiletting has been a constant problem to many staff assisting people with this personal task. There are a number of options that can be considered. The first task is always to adjust the clothing **BEFORE** undertaking the transfer.

The clothing of a heavy or unsteady patient should never be adjusted at the same time as staff are attempting to support the patient's weight.

The options for clothing management are:

Conventional

The person who wears strong cotton knickers of a conventional style can often be supported and rolled from side to side while the skirt is eased up and the knickers are eased down over the person's hips.

The nurse stands in front of the patient with her legs braced against and outside the patient's knees. The patient is supported by the nurse placing one arm around the shoulders and gently pulling the patient slightly forward and to the side being supported. With the free hand, the nurse pulls the skirt up so that it will be clear from underneath the seated person. The roll is then reversed so that the other side is then eased up. After the skirt is clear, then the side to side roll is continued but this time the waist-band of the knickers is pulled down until they are clear of the hips. Several rolls on each side may be required to get both sets of clothing clear of the hips.

Drop Front

These can be made by a very simple clothing adaptation. All women's knickers have a reinforced gusset. The front edge of this gusset is cut across and the two edges rejoined with a strip of appropriately coloured velcro. The 'hook' part of the Velcro faces away from the patient and the soft 'loop' side can then be pressed into place against the patient. This type of design can be used by those people who are wheelchair-bound and who wish to avoid transfer. They can wheel themselves (or be wheeled) into the WC cubicle. Lift the skirt, pull down the adapted gusset and place a hand-held urinal in place or use a funnel and tube over into the WC bowl.

Teddy

A commercially available design of all-in-one, camisole and knickers called a 'teddy' can also serve in the same way as the previously described adaptation. The fastenings on the 'teddy' may need strengthening or enlarging to make access easier.

Legged

For older ladies who like a legged-knicker design, an adaptation can be made which splits the back but

allows full cover and dignity in front. To use this type, the person is again rocked but the knicker is pulled to one side with the waist-band left in place.

Toilet Transfers

Using a Hoist

Wherever the patient requires to be transferred on to a commode or WC and he is non weight-bearing, then the use of a hoist must be considered. There may not be enough floor space in a WC cubicle to use a mobile hoist but there is either the possibility of installing an overhead electric track run hoist or of using a mobile hoist in a more spacious area to move the patient on to a mobile sanichair which is then pushed over the WC (**Fig. 72**). Where there are many dependent people (such as in a residential home) then the use of the overhead electric hoist may be preferred.

Fig 72 *Mobile hoist*

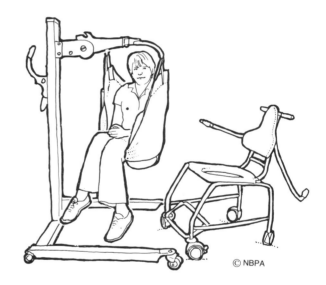

© NBPA

In using either hoist it is important to see first that the hoist and its appropriate attachments are near to hand, the sanichair (if used) is made ready; and privacy is ensured. Secondly, to adjust the patient's clothing so that nothing impedes the toiletting process. If the patient is wearing protective pads (perhaps in special pants) then it may be easier to adjust clothing while lying on a bed or changing couch. The hoist is used to transfer him from the wheelchair to the bed. When the pad is removed and the clothing adjusted, the hoist is again used to place him on a sanichair, commode or the WC. To replace pads and pants, he is again rested on the bed or couch.

Several hoist manufacturers have now developed slings which are particularly designed to assist with toiletting. These slings are often in two pieces. The top sling wraps around the chest of the patient, sometimes with a Velcro fastening. The separate leg sling(s) are placed beneath the patient's thighs. This design allows the nurse to use the hoist to lift the weight of the patient and yet leaves the clothing around the hips and waist free from the sling, allowing the nurse to pull up a skirt and adjust knickers or to remove trousers and underpants (**Fig. 73**).

Fig 73 *Toiletting sling*

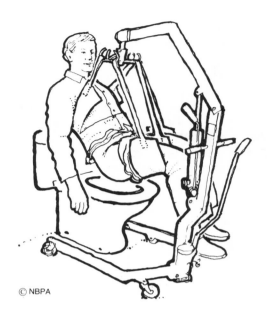

© NBPA

There are several products commercially available which are designed specifically to lift patients to transfer them for toiletting purposes. Most of these products require some cooperation from the patient who must be able to take some weight while being supported in a semi-standing position. The Mobil-aid, the LIC Lifting Stool and more widely used Sara from Arjo-Mecanaids are all useful.

The Sara has a sheepskin covered sling which is placed across the lower part of the patient's back and forward under his axillae. The patient's feet have previously been placed on the footrest of the hoist and his knees positioned close to the knee pad on the hoist mast. The sling is attached to the front arms of the spreader bar and is tensioned. The bar is then lifted by winding a handle on the back of the hoist mast. The patient is raised into a semi-upright position where his clothing can be adjusted before being sat either on the toilet, or on the toilet seat attachment or on a mobile sanichair. Once toiletting is completed, the patient can be raised for cleansing and clothing readjustment before being placed back in his own chair. An advantage of this system is that the patient has the sensation of standing even though he is unable to weight-bear independently.

Manual Transfers

There are various techniques suitable for transferring a patient on and off the toilet. In deciding which approach to take, first ascertain whether the patient can bear weight through his legs and assess the weight which the nurse(s) are likely to lift.

If the patient can weight-bear, is not obese, and can assist with the transfer, then one nurse could use a pelvic or waist-belt hold (particularly if a lifting belt is used as the clothes would have been adjusted for toiletting) or an axillary hold, using a rocking technique.

Elbow Lift Hold

A further technique which is particularly useful for a toilet transfer is the Elbow Lift Hold (**Fig. 74**). This can be used in a confined space and is easily carried out by a nurse who is tall enough for the patient. The patient is positioned on his wheelchair beside the toilet so that the front edges of the two seated areas are adjoining and at a slight angle. The nurse stands in front of the sitting patient, with the foot furthest from the toilet placed in a forward position, the foot nearest the toilet is placed level with the patient's feet and blocking his knees. She should feel stable and able to move her weight freely from one foot to the other. She encourages or helps the patient to lean forwards from his hips so that his near shoulder is firmly against her trunk. She then leans across his back and grasps the outside of his elbows with her fingers beneath them. To prevent his trunk from rotating during the transfer, she locks his far shoulder by bringing her arm in front of it. This grip gives excellent control of the patient's movement. It should be comfortable for the patient with no pressures being exerted on his head or neck:

Fig 74 *Elbow lift hold*

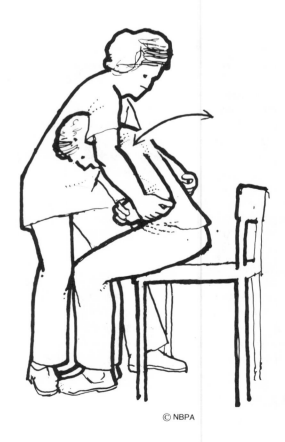

© NBPA

for a confused patient may find it disorientates him if he cannot see where he is going because his head is tipped down and forward. The nurse, having checked that all is ready, then gently rocks the patient towards her several times until a rhythm is established. At a given signal, while the patient is in the forward raised position, the nurse then swings the patient round to place him down on the adjacent toilet seat.

This technique may also be used by two nurses where clothing has to be adjusted, a soiled pad removed and the patient cleansed. One nurse places herself in front as described above and the second nurse is behind the seated patient. The nurse behind the patient can pull down clothing, remove pads and wipe clean as each swing forward raises the patient's hips from the seat. Although this involves the nurse in a reaching movement, it is not a sustained hold and there is minimal lifting.

The principles of rocking a patient before a transfer may be applied to several hand holds.

Manual Lift for Two Nurses Toiletting a Patient

These types of manual transfers should now be approached with extreme caution. It is probable that the weight of the patient, the space available and the task of sitting on a toilet will all contribute to this being a hazardous activity. If the patient is lightweight i.e. 112 lb, (50 kg) and the toilet cubicle has been designed with adequate clear floor space around the toilet pedestal, then it might be possible to use a two nurse manual lift. The techniques possible are all described in the section on bed to chair transfers (Chapter 12).

Chapter 15
Washing and Bathing

Introduction

The choice of methods by which patients are bathed needs to take into account the level of dependency and the assistance which may be required. Only the fittest of patients should be allowed to enter and leave the bath while on their feet.

Lifting a patient manually out of the bath is extremely dangerous and should only be necessary in an emergency. If the patient is taken ill and becomes helpless, then consideration must be given to treating the patient in the bath first, before any stressful and hazardous manual lift is contemplated.

Under no circumstance should the patient be manually lifted from the bath as a routine procedure.

The risks associated with this bathing activity must be carefully assessed. No patient who is unpredictable, obese or known as medically unstable should be allowed to enter a bath without a hoist to retrieve him.

Emergency Procedures

In an emergency, it helps if the water is kept in the bath, partly because it keeps the patient warm, but mainly because the water gives the patient buoyancy.

When the bath is located against a wall, the nurse must be prepared to step into the bath, leaving shoes on or off depending on which option is the least slippery. The Through-arm Grip is probably the most suitable, one foot being in the bath close behind the seated patient and the other outside firmly on the floor. If another nurse is present to assist with lifting the legs of the patient, then both feet in the bath may be more comfortable for the through-arm lifter. The nurse taking the weight of the legs will find that a towel slipped under the patient's mid to upper thighs will give a firm non-slip hold and will prevent the nurse having to stoop in order to secure her hold on wet and slippery legs. If the lift can be planned so that it takes place in several stages then this will reduce some of the truncal stress for the lifter. A number of items such as an inverted washing up bowl or two folded blankets can be used as a halfway stage in the lift. Two smaller lifts, one from the floor of the bath to the temporary seat and then up to the rim of the bath will ease some of the stress on the lifter. The aim is to get the patient high enough to sit him on the edge of the bath so that the legs can be swung over; and then on to a chair or trolley according to circumstances.

When there is access to both sides of the bath, a hoist or smaller item of equipment to assist with bath transfers should always be used. Again this procedure should only be used in emergencies when the patient must be moved from the bath. If the patient is able to hold his own wrists, two nurses may be able to use a modified Through-arm Grip, one on each side, using their other arms as a supporting strut, as with the Shoulder Lift. If a bath seat or other temporary seat is positioned behind the patient, this will enable the lift to be done in two stages.

The single-handed nurse in the community, when faced with a patient unable to get out of the bath, may have to call the ambulance service. Thereafter the nurse will have to resort to bed-baths or a wash-down while the patient is seated, if no bathing equipment has been provided and the patient remains at risk. Likewise this approach must be adopted by hospital nursing staff when the bath and bathroom have not been designed for the use of equipment or when a bath hoist has yet to be provided.

Bath Bench, Seat and Mat

The simplest items of equipment are the bath bench (**Fig. 75**), bath seat and the non-slip bath mat. These three must be used together if the patient is to lower himself into the water. By using these items, the patient may be able to manage his bathing independent of nursing assistance, only supervision being required.

Fig 75 *Bath bench*

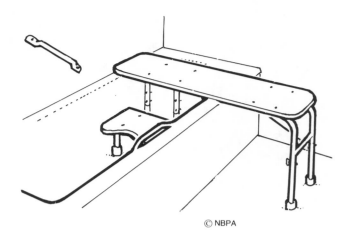

© NBPA

The patient must be able to take his weight through his arms and maintain a good sitting posture. This method is not suitable for people who have arthritic, painful shoulders and elbows since they will find that the stress on their joints while lifting themselves out of the water is uncomfortable. The patient must also be able to move his legs over the side of the bath, with or without some assistance. It is also to be expected that even if an elderly patient can manage his system when he is first referred for help, it should be reviewed regularly to ensure that he is still able to lift his own weight. The bathing equipment should be reviewed and changed, thus avoiding the possibility of the patient becoming stuck, weakened by the effort or in too much pain to move.

Types of Bath Bench and Bath Seat

The bath bench is available in a variety of surfaces and designs. Some have wood or cork surfaces other are plastic or padded plastic for comfort. There are some benches designed with additional drainage holes on the surface to use with a shower over the bath. The advantage of these is that the patient can continue to have a good wash down while sitting over the bath, or to have a shower while seated. The bath or shower bench should fit across the width of the bath and not protrude over the edge unless supported on legs. There are adjustable edges beneath the board to fit against the bath sides and so prevent it from moving as the transfer takes place.

The bath seat has many different designs. Some are small plastic stools with rubber suction feet which can be placed on the floor of the bath. These are available in several heights so that one can be chosen that is about halfway from the top rim to the floor of the bath. Over-bath seats may fit with an adjustable wedging system to secure them against the bath walls but they can only be used with a steel bath or baths of a similarly strong construction. Many people in the community have acrylic or plastic baths which cannot stand the pressure of seat supports against the side walls. A bath seat with side arms that suspend from the rim of the bath must then be chosen. The non-slip bath mat must be placed in front of the seat so that

the patient's feet do not slip as he tries to use them to assist himself back up and out of the bath. Finally, it is possible to alter the height of a bath. Many are set on a frame which can be altered to raise or lower the height of the bath rim. The height of the bath rim must be suitable for a patient to sit and rise unassisted if possible.

Use of the Bath Bench, Seat and Mat

Having prepared for his bath and sat on the board, the patient can lift his legs over the side of the bath, with assistance if necessary and move along the board until he is sitting centrally. By using his arms he can lift himself from the board down on to the bath seat. If the bath is of sufficient length, the patient may then lift himself again to the floor of the bath. Many patients will, however, stay on the bath seat, half submerged in the bath water, to wash themselves and soak their legs. A non-slip mat under the patient's feet will help him push with his legs to move from the floor of the bath to the seat and from the seat to the bench. Once up on the bench, the patient's legs can be swung over the bath rim and he can be dried while sitting on the bath board. But when elderly patients find it difficult or painful to push up on their arms, the bathing procedure should be reviewed.

Bath Hoists

There are four different types of hoist to assist a patient in and out of the bath. The choice will depend on the design and space within the bathroom and on the mobility and support needs of the patient who is to use it.

Internal Bath Hoists

These are bath hoists which fit inside the bath and take up no additional space. Several are available, operating through compressed air, sealed electrical battery power or by mechanical levers. Before placing such a hoist in the base of the bath, it is wise to remove the side bath panel and check the construction. In the case of lightweight bath material, it may be advisable to place supportive blocks of wood beneath the section of the bath floor where the hoist will be placed.

Those bath hoists that use an air compressor (**Fig. 76**), require the compressor to be operated from a power point outside the bathroom and only the air line from the compressor unit should enter the bathroom. The hand control to operate such a bath hoist is a simple on/off switch to open or close the supply of air which inflates the bellows below the bath hoist seat. Some bath hoists operate through sealed electrical battery packs which are usually fastened on the top of the seat design or in the hand held control. These have proved to be easy to use and recharge.

The points to consider when choosing such an internal hoist reflect both the abilities of the patient

Fig 76 *Internal bath hoist using compressed air*

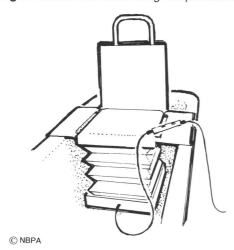

© NBPA

who uses it and the other people who may use the same bathroom. The patient must be able to sit on the bath hoist seat and move his legs over the rim of the bath. This is a similar movement to the use of the bath board and seat. However, the strain of lifting body weight is taken from the patient and the hoist will raise and lower him into the water. If other people use the bathroom, then leaving the bath hoist in position may be beneficial to other patients. However, in the community, some family members may not wish to use the bath with the hoist in position. The difficulty of lifting the hoist in and out of the bath must be considered. Most bath hoists have large suction cups on the hoist feet so that they can be firmly fixed to the bath base. To lift the hoist from the bath, these four suction feet have to be released while the weight of the hoist is balanced at an angle. This is awkward and not easy for a carer who may already be under stress. The noise of the hoist motor or air compressor may also be a factor which influences some people's choice. Bathrooms are sometimes resonant rooms and the noise from an electric motor may be too penetrating for some patients. The other considera- tion which must be discussed with patients is whether or not the patient wishes to lie down in the bath or at least to lie back for a good long soak. It may be this long warm soak which is considered the most therapeutic attribute of a bath and therefore it will be important to the patient how much of his body can be immersed. Very few of these types of bath hoist allow the patient to lie back in the water.

External Bath Hoists

This type of bath hoist is mounted on a pillar external to the bath (**Fig. 77**) and often has a detachable seat which can be used on a mobile chassis. This pillar mounting requires additional floor space within the bathroom and the construction of the floor needs to be checked; not all concrete construction floors are suitable for this type of installation. The pillar mount- ing may have a brake on it to stabilise the hoist seat during transfers. The seat may have an extended leg piece which will help the single-handed nurse both to operate the hoist and manoeuvre the patient's legs over the side of the bath. It is the detachable seat and

chassis which most patients find useful. The seat, on its chassis, can be wheeled to the bedroom and the patient transferred on to it. The mobile unit and the patient can then be wheeled over a toilet or into a treatment room before reaching the bathroom. Once the patient is prepared for the bath, his chair unit is attached to the pillar, the chassis is detached and the chair swung over the bath and down into the water.

When considering this type of bath hoist, the floor space may dictate where the hoist pillar is positioned and it is possible to get a mounting that can be used either at the side or at the end of the bath.

Mobile Hoists

There are three main types of mobile hoist for bathroom use and for each of them a large bathroom is required with space to manoeuvre the hoist. First the mobile hoist which is normally used for other transfers may also be used for bath transfers if a channel has been cut in the lower edge of the bath side panel so that the legs of the hoist chassis can pass beneath the floor of the bath.

Secondly, some mobile hoists have an additional socket which can be mounted on the bathroom floor. The mast of the mobile hoist can be removed and replaced in the floor socket. This might be useful in the community, where a range of transfers in one house create a need for several items of lifting equipment.

Thirdly, some mobile bath hoists are available which have been designed to assist a patient from the bed, transport him to the bathroom and then assist him in a bath or a shower area. The patient stays sitting on it throughout and must have enough postural control to do this.

Fig 77 *External bath hoist*

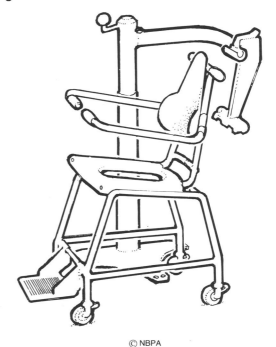

© NBPA

For patients with poor postural control the hoist seat is unsuitable and slings should be used. Both wet and dry slings will be needed and the number required for different patients' needs must be reviewed.

All too often a large mobile hoist is found in the bathroom but it is rarely used outside that room. Space and costs can be saved if more mobile hoists are used on the ward and more static bath hoists are used in the bathroom.

Overhead Electric Hoists

Where space is at a premium but a bath transfer system is needed, an overhead track with an electric hoist motor should provide a safe bath handling procedure (Fig. 78). The hoists use low-voltage and are safe in bathroom areas. The newer models are without trailing power cables and there is a wide range of sling designs to suit all types of patients needs.

Bathroom Design

There are two basic bathroom designs; the first where the long side of the bath is against a wall and the second where the bath juts out into the room with space on both sides. In the community, the bath is most often against the wall and the choice of bath hoist has to take into account the use of the bathroom by other family members. In the hospital ward, the choice between the two designs may be affected by the assistance which the nurse has to give the patient being bathed. It is better to be able to reach both sides of the patient without too much stretching and stooping.

The tasks which have to be completed within a bathroom must be considered, so that appropriate space can be created for them. Patients will often get undressed and dressed within the bathroom. The nurse assisting a patient to dry himself and to dress, will require not only space around the wheelchair or bath hoist chair, but also places to leave clothes, towels and other bathroom items within reach. The stooped working postures that are often adopted by the nurse lead to cumulative back strain and can be easily prevented by careful planning of the working environment.

One of the greatest hazards in the bathroom area is that of the wet floor. Floor materials must be non-slip and nurses should take extra care over the selection of suitable supportive non-slip footwear to use in the bathroom. If a bathroom has been used for one patient and water spilled on the floor, then it should be wiped and dried before the next patient is taken to be bathed.

The Design of the Bath

The height of the bath, as well as its construction, can do much to make the bath easy to use by any patient.

Fig 78 *Electric overhead hoist*

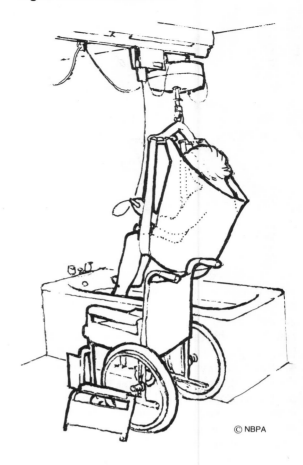

© NBPA

The bath rim should be of a height which allows patients to sit and rise easily if a bath board and seat are being used. There are adjustable height baths which allow the bath to be lowered to assist the patient in and then raised to allow the nurse to help without stooping. If these are used in conjunction with a hoist, then the whole bathing task becomes a much safer activity for both patient and nurse. There is also a height adjustable bath which is mobile with a fold down side panel enabling it to be used as a changing bench for patients who are incontinent.

There are moulded baths with a removable side panel which allows the patient to slide across onto an internal seat. The panel is replaced and the bath can be tipped slightly backwards so that the 'greater proportion of the patient's body is immersed in warm water. When choosing such a specialist design of bath, it is important to check how the patient is expected to enter and leave the bath. If it cannot be used with a hoist and dependent patients are to use it, then alternatives should be sought.

Sit-baths have been popular over the years and a number of different designs are still available. Some mobile bath hoists have been developed to transport the patient, and while still seated to be enclosed within the bath cabinet. Others require the patient to stand and step into the cabinet before the door is sealed and the water added. To assist with this transfer, some manufacturers have designed a mobile seat so that the patient stands, turns around and sits on a seat which is then pushed back into the cabinet before the door is sealed in place. While these types of designs might be useful for the confused patient or those who lack confidence to enter a full bath, they create some postural problems for the nurse who is assisting the patient to wash. The sides of the cabinet and the door are above the waist height and the assisting nurse has to lean over them to reach the patient. The patient's feet and legs are best left until the water has been released and the door can be opened. The nurse can then squat down to reach into the footwell of the bath.

Neither the baths with removable side-panels nor the sit-baths are suitable for patients who have to be transferred with manual assistance.

Showers

Showers are often thought to be the answer when patients have extreme mobility problems and bathing becomes difficult. Without careful consideration, the wrong choice of shower tray and fitting could also deny the patient access to a full body wash in comfort and privacy. It should be borne in mind when planning a patient's care or selecting a shower system, that falls in the shower are not uncommon and a patient who is unsteady puts both himself and the nurse at risk.

There are five different ways in which a shower can be installed and the needs of various patients will determine which is the most suitable.

Shower Trays

Shower trays come in a number of different sizes, usually square but sometimes oblong. The problem with a shower tray is that the user has to step over the rim. If there is already a mobility problem (which is why a shower is being considered) then this difficulty could lead to the shower being rejected. The other difficulty for people with stiff joints is that when they sit on the shower seat, their legs protrude forwards over the rim of the tray, pushing the shower curtain out and thus allowing water to spread over the bathroom floor. The use of a shower tray also excludes the use of a mobile shower chair.

Flat Access Shower

A shower providing flat access will allow a mobile shower tray to be used. Many disabled people may choose to transfer from bed to shower chair and then go straight to the bathroom to use the toilet and shower; this facility avoids the need for several transfers and may allow the hoist to be used in the bedroom only. The shower base may be a pre-moulded platform which is set into the floor, or a quarry tiled floor is provided with a very slight slope into the drain in one corner of the wet area. This design allows a variety of patients to use their own seating or support system while washing. Care should be taken to ensure, before installation, that drainage will be adequate as showers quickly fall into disuse if flooding occurs.

Shower over the Bath or Toilet

If space is limited and in the community there are family considerations, then providing a shower over a bath with a shower bench across the bath may be one solution. The patient has to be able to transfer on and off the seat and to get his legs over the rim of the bath. There is a modified type of bath seat which fits on two struts across the bath. The seat on this frame can be turned at 90° so that the patient can back up to it and sit, the seat then turns around while his feet are lifted across the bath rim. This seat gives greater support than a bench and is excellent when the patient is trying to bend and wash himself and needs a more stable base.

In the community, it may be possible to provide a downstairs toilet but where there is not enough space for a bathroom or shower-room as well, it is possible for a shower to be fitted over the toilet. The WC becomes the shower seat and if the toilet is fully tiled it becomes a multiple-use area.

Shower Cubicles

Where a shower area is being created but space is short, shower cubicles may be considered. These can be placed in a corner of the bathroom, can replace a bath or sometimes can be sited within the patient's bedroom. They consist of a waterproof base with high sides, and sometimes a top roof cover. The entry wall often has a stable door design so that a carer can assist. Some models have lower sides all around so that access can be obtained by the carer from the sides as well as from the front. The cubicle may have a seat or may be ramped to allow a mobile shower chair to be used within it. Generally these shower cubicles are most suitable for those patients who are able to help themselves, as the postural stress incurred by nurses and carers who have to stoop, stretch and reach to assist the patient is exhausting. One type of cubicle, suitable for patients who can transfer from a wheelchair with minimal assistance provides for all needs including toiletting and showers and can be sited in a bedroom.

Shower Trolleys

A final system to consider is that of the mobile shower trolley which may have a padded insert for the comfort of the dependent user. These trolleys can be adjustable in height and can be wheeled to the patient's bedside. An Easislide (Chapter 10) may be used to move the adult patient from his bed to the trolley, and then he is wheeled through to the shower area. The showering and drying of the patient is all done at the height most suitable for the nurse, usually just above the waist height (Fig. 79). This lessens the amount of reaching and stooping which thus reduces the stress on the nurse. This type of equipment is in frequent use where there are a number of high dependency patients. The padded inserts to the trolley are suitable when epilepsy or other uncontrollable body movements may mean the patient could injure himself. The side of the trolley can be lowered to ease the side transfer of the patient.

Fig 79 *Shower trolley*

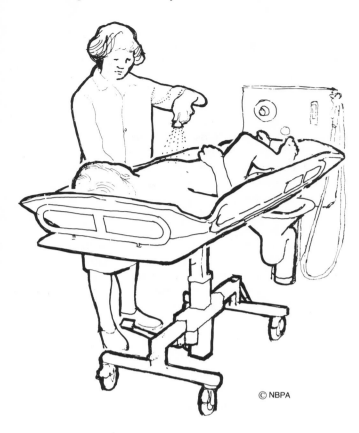

© NBPA

Fig 80 *Small mobile hoist*

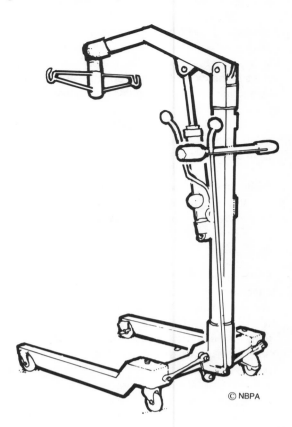

© NBPA

The Choices Available

With the variety of bathing and washing alternatives, it should also be possible to select a method which offers both comfort and privacy to the patient and a comfortable working posture for the nurse. Costs may be much reduced by selecting the right option. The provision of a bath hoist (**Fig. 80**) will be considerably cheaper than the renovation of an existing bathroom to convert it to a shower room. Many patients prefer a long hot soak to a shower, where they can easily become cold while wet. Several hospital units for long-stay patients are also finding the use of a spa bath, much on the same style as a jacuzzi, to be very beneficial for many patients. The action of the water

and air bubbles against the skin promotes good circulation. This aids healing, and relaxes as well as cleanses the patient.

Bathing and washing is one of the most strenuous tasks for nurses to perform and care must be taken to reduce this stress whenever possible. If none of the alternatives described above can be supplied or are unsuitable for either the nurse or the patient, then a strip wash or a bed bath must always be considered. Apart from nurses, carers at home such as the mother with a disabled child, will find that a bath insert to support the small patient may assist in alleviating stress. The difficulties of both supporting and washing a patient are back-threatening and should be avoided at all costs.

The Falling Patient

Patients who are at risk of falling should be taught: first, how to fall safely and then how they should rise (see Figure 82).

If while supporting a patient the helper finds that she is starting to bear the weight of the patient and he is about to fall she must not hesitate: it is invariably safer to let the patient down in a controlled manner to the floor. In order to do this she must be at his side and half behind him. With both hands supporting him round the waist, but not joined, she can then pull him back against the top of her thigh nearest to him, shuffle her feet backwards and, using her forearms to protect his head, slide him down her body until he is supported in a seated position against her legs. As she does this she slides her hands up into his axillae and can thus keep her back reasonably erect throughout the procedure (**Figs. 81a, b & c**).

This is a skilled manoeuvre and nurses must be given the opportunity to practice it following demonstration, in order to counteract their natural instincts to save the patient from falling.

If the nurse is some way away from the patient when he starts to fall, she can only break his fall as best she can, getting in behind him if time allows.

Moving a Patient from the Floor

Manual lifting of a patient from the floor is such a high risk activity that assessment of the situation is essential. The key considerations must always be the safety of not only the person on the floor but also the stress on the nurse. The first decision to make concerns the safety of the patient: whether he can be moved or whether treatment should be offered *in situ*. It is possible to attend to a patient in an epileptic state

Figure 81a-c *Supporting the falling patient*

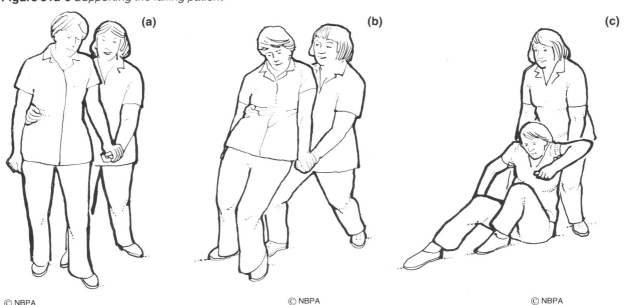

(a)   (b)   (c)

© NBPA   © NBPA   © NBPA

on the floor, or to treat following a cardiac arrest without the unnecessary risk of lifting a body in an unstable or critical condition. The history of the fall will influence the decision to move or not. An observed, or controlled fall, of a known patient will require a different response from that required when entering a house to find someone who may have been on the floor for a long period of time and where the circumstances of the fall are unknown. Once the professional decision to move him has been made, then a number of options are open.

The first task is always to comfort and reassure. It is distressing for the fallen patient who will often be in an anxious and agitated state and urging the nurse to help them up as fast as possible. The nurse must stop and assess the situation before proceeding with help. While this assessment is being made, the patient should be reassured, and his personal comfort and dignity respected. A pillow behind the head (or sitting him up, propped against furniture) will assist him to collect himself and become less anxious. If necessary he should be screened from inquisitive visitors. It may be helpful for another person to sit on the floor with him and calmly reassure him while the assistance is being organised.

Assessment

Always – STOP – THINK !

The assessment process has four components:

The Task

What is the task that has to be done next?
Is the move to be from the floor to bed, to a chair or somewhere else?
What are the heights and distances of the move?
Will a manual lift require the lifter to adopt a bent, stooped, twisted or other awkward position?
Is the patient to be lifted in a stable state or likely to have sudden movements that will make a manual lift uncontrollable?

The Load (the patient)

How heavy is he?
If the manual lift is to be in a stooped or bent position then the share of his weight will be multiplied, sometimes five fold. Is he difficult to grasp because of his body shape or physical difficulties (such as painful joints)?
Can he comprehend and will he follow instructions?
Has he been taught how to roll and crawl to get on to a low chair?
Can he maintain a sitting balance and assist you to move him?

The Environment

Where has he fallen?
How much space is there around him?
Is he in a safe place or in a situation likely to put him at further risk?
Is he hot or cold or in danger of being chilled or overheated?

How well lit is the area both for reassuring the patient and for allowing the nurse to see how help can be given?
Has he fallen in an area where there are steps, stairs, narrow corridors, corners and confined spaces that make lifting him from the floor hazardous?

The Nurse or Carer's Capabilities

What are your qualifications to help the patient in this situation?
Will you need help?
If so how can it be summoned?
Are you in good health?
Will you be at risk yourself?
What are the risks to the patient if you try to manage on your own?
Have you been taught how to approach and move a patient who is found on the floor?
Are there instructions and procedures that should be followed?
How accessible are the written procedures should they need to be checked?
What equipment is at hand to assist with the move and have you been taught how to use this equipment?

The Less Dependent Patient

People who are at risk of falling, such as those who have suffered a stroke or who are afflicted by Parkinson's disease should be taught what to do on falling. This is standard practice in physiotherapy. First, they should be taught how to let themselves down to the floor without harm in the event that they find themselves losing balance. Next they should learn how to get up and how best they can assist the nurse or carer who has come to the rescue. This involves turning over onto their knees, then into a half-kneeling posture with one foot flat on the floor, ready to push themselves up onto the adjacent chair (Fig. 82). A belt firmly fastened round the patient's waist will assist the carer to manoeuvre him into position.

Fig 82 *Patient getting up from floor as taught.*

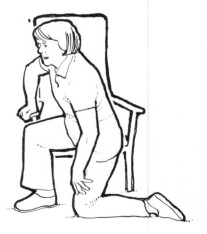

© NBPA

The Dependent Patient

Moving an adult patient who cannot assist requires the use of a hoist. Where the lift is from the floor, then a hoist is the only safe method. All manual methods involve stooped and awkward postures and the risk of injury.

Before the hoist and sling are located and brought into position, the patient may first have to be slid into an area to create more space around him in which to use the hoist (see next section on sliding sheets etc). He is then helped to a sitting position by propping him against the bed or an upturned chair with pillow to soften the support (Fig. 83a).

The hoist sling, preferably of a divided leg design, is positioned around the patient (Fig. 83b). First, the nurse pulls him forward so that she can place the sling across his back and tuck it down to the buttock crease before easing him back on to the pillows. She should then check that the sling has been centrally placed and is supporting the shoulders. The two leg pieces are pulled forwards, one on either side. Checking that they are not twisted, gently he is rolled slightly to one side so that the leg part of the sling can be eased under the buttocks. The other side is treated the same. The leg pieces are then pulled forward and taken under each leg so that they cross beneath the knees. Check that the leg pieces are as close to the knees as possible; and flat, thus preventing pressure from creases in the fabric. Sometimes it is necessary to use the hoist to take up tension in order to straighten out any creases. The patient is then ready to be lifted in the hoist.

If the only sling available is a one-piece sling without divided legs, the patient may have to be rolled to get it into position. But if the patient is still feeling dizzy, beware of too much movement.

The hoist may be positioned in one of two ways depending on where the space is best used. If the space is at the side of the patient then the hoist chassis may approach from the side with one chassis leg under his crooked knees and the other leg in the space between his buttocks and the propping chair and pillows.

If the space is at the patient's feet, then the hoist approaches from the feet with one chassis leg either side of him. If he has long legs, it may be necessary to place an extra cushion or pillow on the back of the hoist chassis to protect his ankles and shins.

In either hoist position, the chassis is manoeuvred to bring the centre of the spreader bar close to the patient's hips so that a straight lift can be achieved. This may involve lowering the boom of the hoist as far as possible. The straps on the sling can then be attached. The shoulder attachments should be as tight as possible and on the highest point of suspension; while the leg sling attachments are fastened at the longest point of suspension. Where an Ambulift

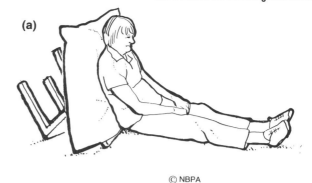

(a)

© NBPA

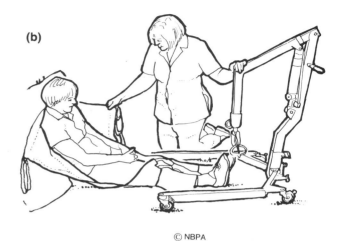

(b)

© NBPA

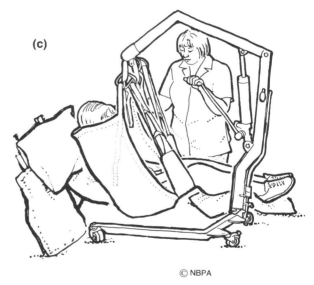

(c)

© NBPA

Fig 83a-c *Moving a dependent patient from the floor*

model D is used, the sling bar attachment may need to be lowered in order to facilitate the attachment of the sling loops. This should enable the patient to be lifted in a sitting position, ready to be placed in a chair or on the bed.

Having checked the sling attachments and ensured that the legs of the hoist are not on top of the sling, the nurse then operates the hoist to lift the patient (Fig. 83c). It is helpful at this moment if she is kneeling on the floor so that she can maintain eye contact with the patient as well as keeping a reassuring hand in place as the lift commences. As he is lifted, she can pause in the operation of the hoist to get herself to her feet before the patient reaches the required height of lift. It may then be necessary to move any pillows around the chassis before moving the hoist to the chair or bed.

It is possible to undertake this procedure with one nurse but two people maybe required, particularly when the patient remains distressed and disoriented.

This procedure is also recommended wherever and whenever the dependent person is on the floor by design. Many people have to be cared for on the floor either for safety or for purposes of treatment; for example:

- adults with multiple handicaps who may use bean bags or soft play mats on the floor as part of their free movement, stretching and therapeutic exercise-regime.

- elderly dependent people who are suffering from dementia, restlessness and who are likely to damage themselves on bed or cot-sides and who may be nursed on a mattress on the floor.

- patients starting out on their rehabilitation programmes who may still be dependent but who are being taught an exercise regime to increase mobility. These people may be treated by physiotherapists and others on the floor. Lifting a patient from the floor should always involve the use of a hoist until he is able to get up himself with minimal help.

Moving a Lightweight Patient from the Floor to Bed

Where the patient on the floor can co-operate, has sitting balance and is under 112 lb (50 kg) in weight, it may be possible to use one of several items of handling equipment.

The Transit Seat

This is a commercially available nylon canvas seat with reinforced hand-grips (**Fig. 84**). It also has a waist safety strap and has detachable shoulder straps to assist with carrying.

The patient can be can be rolled on to this seat either by a full body roll or by side to side rocking to ease the seat canvas beneath his hips. Two, three or four people can then position themselves and by grasping the hand grips can lift him while maintaining an upright posture.

This Transit seat has been found to be useful to carry older children who are not yet full adult body size but who present significant weights to be handled. Some people have found it useful for carrying children on and off buses; others to carry children up and

Fig 84 *The transit seat*

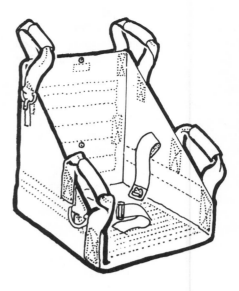

© NBPA

downstairs; or to assist with getting children in and out of swimming pools.

A Lifting Sheet

These are commercially available and come in a variety of sizes. They are made of friction free slippery material which has additional strengthened hand-grips at the corners and around the edges of the sheet.

These sheets are mainly used to reposition people who have fallen in confined spaces or who require to be moved short distances such as up the bed. To place the sheet under a person on the floor they can either be rolled or, if the space or the patient's condition does not permit this, the sheet is folded in a concertina fashion and placed under his head and shoulders. The top edge of the sheet stays level with the top of the head and one assistant kneels or stands astride the patient's head with their knees or feet anchoring the sheet to the floor. A second assistant stands astride the patient's body and grasps the hand-grips on the lower edge of the sheet. Moving away from the patient's head, backwards down the body, a sharp pulling motion will cause the sheet to become unfolded and flattened beneath him. The nurse doing this needs to ensure that she does not twist or attempt to lift while working in this bent position. With two, three or four assistants, the person on the floor can then be pulled into an area where further attention can be given to his treatment or to the lift from the floor.

This sheet can also be used on the bed for a heavy patient who needs to be eased up the bed against the pillows. The use of a friction free sheet beneath his body on the bed will eliminate the need to lift since there will no frictional forces between his skin and the sheet.

Blanket Lift from Floor

Where the patient is lightweight and there is a minimum of four lifters (and preferably six) a traditional Blanket Lift from floor may be used.

The blanket is rolled beneath the patient and, if necessary, a small pillow put under his head. Next, the patient may have to be slid into a favourable position for the lift. This will depend on where the patient is lying, on the space available around the bed and on access to the bed. The bed itself may have to be moved.

> **Under no circumstances should the lifters attempt to lift the patient on to the bed from the side, when the patient is parallel to the bed: it is impossible to do this without major contortions.**

It will be best to slide the patient to the foot of the bed; ready to be lifted on to the end. The six lifters take position with the strongest lifters in the middle for the heaviest share of the lift. The leader gives the word of command: and the patient is lifted first on to the end of the bed where his head and shoulders are rested. After readjusting their positions and holds as necessary, the lifters next take the patient to the centre of the bed; finally placing him in position with his head on the pillows.

The blanket lift should only be undertaken by strong lifters and should be practised under supervision.

Moving a Lightweight Patient from the Floor to Chair

If the patient is lightweight and is able to sit on the floor and co-operate with the nurses, then several other methods may be appropriate and safe to move him to a chair.

Using a Shoulder Lift to Hoist Seat

If there is a hoist available with a seat attachment but no hoist-slings, then this may be used to assist with a lift from the floor. The patient is eased into a sitting position. The hoist is wheeled and placed behind him and the brakes are locked. The seat attachment is lowered to the lowest possible position and the seat arms are swung back.

Two nurses get into a full kneeling position facing the hoist, one on either side of the patient. They place their outside hands forward on the chassis legs of the hoist. They then position themselves with their inside shoulders against the patient's chest wall; using a finger grip, a wrist grip or a towel under the patient's thighs. The patient places his arms over the nurses' shoulders and backs (**Fig. 85**). At a given command, he is lifted the 4″ (100 mm) from the floor on to the hoist seat in either one or two stages until he is in

position on the back of the seat. The arms of the seat are swung forward and, after reassuring him, the hoist mechanism is operated. The patient can either be transported on the hoist or the seat can be lowered on to a mobile chassis, detached from the hoist and the patient then moved in this mobile sanichair. Tall nurses (5′ 8″ (175cm) and upwards) should not attempt this procedure because of the extreme flexion of hips and knees involved. Nurses with limited mobility in hips and knees will also want to avoid this procedure.

Using Improvised Steps

If the patient is lightweight and able to sit and co-operate, it may be possible to create several steps from the floor to a low easy chair. A number of domestic items may serve: a footstool, a pouffe or even some telephone directories. The steps should not be more than about 4″ (100 mm) and should be of a size to take the patient's buttocks.

Having organised the space, the chair and the improvised steps, the two carers can adopt the Shoulder Lift; with a pause to relax between each step.

Handling Policies

In all written policies and procedures on the handling of patients, a clear expectation must be made by the employer about safety of lifting people from the floor.

Some employers state that **NO PERSON** should be lifted manually from the floor and the use of a hoist is mandatory. Where it is left to the nursing and care staff to assess and decide on their methods of handling, there are training implications which must clearly point out the dangers of such practices with all but lightweight people.

Fig 85 *Shoulder lift to hoist seat*

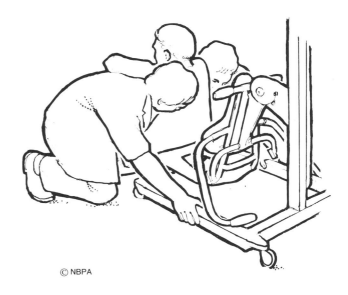

© NBPA

Chapter 17 Special Patient Needs

Lifting and Carrying Children

Children are often not perceived as producing lifting and handling difficulties as they are general considered to be 'lightweight'. However, when caring for children, the posture in which many nurses find themselves can lead to a high level of postural stress and the additional lifting of children, often from the floor will cause and aggravate low back pain.

Anyone who is nursing a child or working with children who have disabilities should check through the following list of precautions:

- Check the height from which you are lifting. Have you prepared the working environment?

- Is the cot-side down and where are you lifting the child to?

- Kneel or squat down to the child's level. Can the child be placed at a higher level to avoid stooping?

- Does the child have any form of disability? Is there any reason for the child not to co-operate and follow verbal instructions if possible?

- If you experience difficulty lifting a particular child, then try to avoid a repetition; reconsider your approach and amend your position.

- Older disabled children can only be safely lifted by using the same approach as for adults. Callipers or support braces, increase the weight, and physical deformities add to the difficulty of the task.

- The child must be carried close to the nurse's trunk (**Fig. 86**). Holding the child in a position so that the back of his head and body are against the lifter follows the principle that the heaviest part of the 'load' is against the lifter's body. This is often a more comfortable position for the child.

- If the lifter is using a body worn sling for a younger child, then it is less stressful for the lifter if the sling is worn on the back rather than the front of their body.

- If the child's body and/or legs tend to go into an extensor spasm, then he is best carried 'folded up' with his hip and knee joints flexed.

Lifting from a Cot

Cots with fixed sides or sides which do not lower right down to mattress level should be rejected as they force the nurse to lift the child with outstretched arms and in a forward stoop. This is a dangerous action. The cot-side should be lowered and the child slid across the mattress towards the nurse. Sometimes the child can be sat up and turned so that his back is towards the nurse or moved onto his front (**Fig. 87**). The lift can then follow the principles of holding the 'load' close to the lifter's body. Where treatment or other tasks cause the nurse to work in a forward flexed position because the mattress level of the cot is too low, then methods of raising the height of the cot, or of changing its design, should be sought.

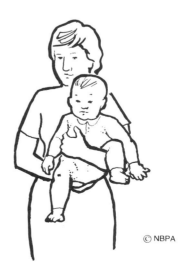

© NBPA

Fig 86 *Holding child with heaviest part of the 'load' against the lifter's body*

Fig 87 *Lifting a child from a cot*

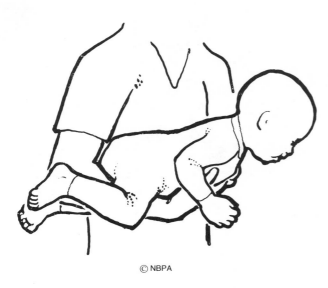

© NBPA

Fig 88a&b *Lifting a child from the floor*

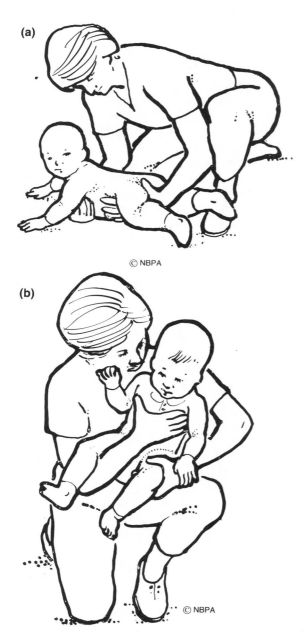

(a)

© NBPA

(b)

© NBPA

Lifting from a Pushchair.

The nurse must kneel on one or both knees to ensure that she is at the level of the pushchair seat and the child. In this lower position she can adjust and fasten safety straps and attend to the child. To lift the child out, he is edged forward on to the nurse's knee before the nurse stands upright.

Lifting from the Floor

When the child is lying on the floor, the nurse kneels down beside the child and places one arm between the child's legs with the palm of the nurse's hand on the child's stomach (**Fig. 88a**). The other hand is placed under the child at shoulder level. The child is rolled towards the nurse so that his back is nearest the nurse. If the nurse presses her hand against the child's stomach, he will flex and bend his hips thus making it easier to lift him (**Fig. 88b**). The hand on the child's shoulder is slid down and round so that it holds the child's thigh while still supporting his body on her forearm. While bending the child's leg towards the nurse she can lift the child on to her lap. The nurse can then rise to stand.

In many instances, older children, particularly those who are profoundly handicapped, are placed on the floor either for play, treatment, exercise or for relaxation. This situation must now be regarded as potentially stressful for the nurse and staff who have to lift the child to and from the floor. Alternative methods should be sought to manual handling. Either a hoist should be used for all floor lifts or the child is not placed so low on the ground. Raised plinths and couches with safety features such as padded sides may be used instead.

The Patient who is Unwilling to Co-operate

This section sets out some basic principles which nurses need to bear in mind when faced with a patient who for a variety of reasons may not be a willing partner in the transfer.

There are specific groups of patients to whom these principles particularly apply. These may be summarised as:

- People with learning disabilities.

- People with acute mental health needs.

- People with organic dementias and disorders characterised by disorientation.

- People who are violent, disorientated or disturbed due to substance abuse, alcohol or drugs.

- People who are violent due to a personality problem.

Duty of Care

A nurse has a basic duty of care to her patient or client. She has to be responsive to the patient's needs and provide competent care at all times. In meeting this challenge the nurse must be aware of and observe the following precautions:

- The nurse should ensure that she has had specific instructions in the principles and practices of handling techniques applicable to the client group concerned.

- The nurse should be both confident and competent in her ability to handle clients in safety for any of the client groups identified. There needs to be a statement to that effect in the training record.

- The ward manager and or team leader must also assess the competence of the nurse and be fully aware of the nurse's skills both in handling and managing such patients.

In fulfilling this responsibility, the ward manager/team leader should assess the competence of the nurse in:

- Her ability, to communicate effectively with the patient.

- Her assertion skills in declaring her right as a practitioner to decide whether or not to become immediately involved in any situation.

- Her risk assessment skills. This implies that the nurse can take a calculated course of action following an assessment of the situation consistent with the available resources and the urgency of the situation.

In meeting these criteria, nurses have a responsibility to exercise judgement. The nurse should wait rather than rush in as a matter of principle. The nurse should seek to calm a situation, adopt an encouraging and reassuring manner and call for or await the arrival of help.

It is the duty of the institution to ensure that adequate help is readily available when this is needed and called for.

The overriding rule is that nurses dealing with aggressive or unco-operative patients should not place themselves at risk any more than nurses in any other situation.

Handling Skills Required for the Confused or Frightened Patient

Confusion, fear and aggression are closely interlinked and each state may present the nurse with a handling problem. This is usually found in the patient who has difficulty in co-operating and tends to struggle or react against the carer involuntarily. The skill, one of the most challenging in nursing, is to enable this person to feel calm and safe, and in a mood to help. Sometimes this might mean leaving

him alone for a while; at other times nothing more than a confident tone of voice, or even just a smile; or yet again, a particular way of holding him which makes him feel the nurse is with him, not against him. There are no rules for this situation, only principles and empathy.

A person who is not able to behave or think logically is extra sensitive to mood and non-verbal signals coming from other people. If his carer is tense or nervous, he also is likely to feel tense and his fears may come to the surface, possibly resulting in aggression. Even if he only stiffens up he will be more difficult to handle. The first principle then is to relax, and assume a confidence that may not be felt. When the patient starts to relax and co-operate, confidence will increase.

People who are deeply anxious sometimes feel they are being 'crowded'. This makes them want to hit out. Their need for space must be respected. Other people who are frightened need the reassurance of a kindly touch, which means more to them than words.

Confusion and fear may be caused simply by sensory loss and disorientation. The nurse can make a handling task easier for herself by ensuring that her patient knows where he is and what is expected of him; that he can see the chair that he is being moved to; that he understands, from instruction clearly and quietly repeated, in which direction he is to turn or where he is to put his hands.

Some flooring can create fearful visual impressions. To a disorientated mind, the space in a ward can seem so immense as to be impassable and big blocks of colour may appear as barriers which stop the patient in his tracks, while a very gentle slope may seem like a precipice.

A person who is in pain or frightened needs to be given as much control of his own movements as possible: encourage him to take the initiative; **invite** him to stand up, or turn over. An elderly lady with learning disabilities who was going blind and becoming unmanageable in her residential home appeared to be unable to move at all on admission to hospital and nurses found it very difficult to stand her up. Enquiries at the home obtained the information that she had been ambulant until that week, but seemed frightened because she could not see. The next morning the nurse asked this lady if she would like to walk with her out to the toilet. The patient stood up, took her hand and walked out with her – thus a patient-handling problem was averted. But the nurse knows only too well that some patients respond best to a voice of authority. So, there are no rules, but it is essential that a sensitive assessment of the patient's capabilities and responses is made and useful information recorded in the Care Plan.

A 'confrontational' approach tends to set up resistance from a confused or frightened patient, while with the 'indirect' approach the patient feels the sympathetic touch of the nurse's hands on his skin and by reflex responses 'gathers' himself in the intended direction of movement before any actual lift is attempted. But if there is any threat of hurt or sense of being outnumbered his reflex response will be in the opposite direction, away from the nurses.

When helping these patients to move, the nurse should position herself very close to give a feeling of security (Fig. 89). If he is frightened of walking and tends to lean backwards, the nurses, one on either side can hold his forearms resting on their own forearms, tucked in to rest on their hips. Patients should be encouraged and reminded about taking their weight through their feet, so avoiding a backward lean. In this way the patient feels totally secure and supported, and the nurses are taking his weight through their legs, minimising any strain.

If the patient has to be lifted manually in or out of bed, a feeling of security can also be transmitted by the use of the Cross-arm Lift (see Figure 59) while the Shoulder Lift is less suitable for a frightened patient who may feel very vulnerable perched on top of the nurses' backs.

The heavy, dependent patient for whom a mobile hoist is called for, may, initially need reassurance. Though the hoist offers a very comfortable and safe mode of transfer, it may not look like it to the patient: he may be scared of it. The first experience of the hoist must therefore be good. The time taken to overcome any fears will be well spent.

Handling Skills Required for the Maliciously Aggressive Patient

This guide does not address the issue of control and restraint of violent or aggressive patients who are detained in security institutions. This section, however, deals with the patient who may be confused, irrational or malicious.

Such patients may withhold their co-operation intentionally from the outset of a handling task or during it. The patient may attack the nurse by biting, scratching, deliberately falling or throwing their weight onto the nurse. Other problems known to arise are caused when the patient lifts his feet off the floor and swings on the nurses arms. This is particularly likely to happen if the nurses are using the Drag Hold, e.g. with the nurses' forearms under the patient's armpits.

All handling tasks involving such patients require the nurse to proceed with considerable caution if the nurse is to avoid injury. If the handling technique is likely to be uncomfortable the patient may resent being handled. For these reasons whenever an aggressive, confused, irrational or malicious patient is to be handled the procedure should be carefully considered and planned beforehand.

The nurse should keep the patient under close supervision at all times.

Fig 89 *Walking a confused patient – with one nurse*

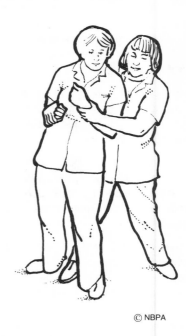

© NBPA

Fig 90a *Walking an aggressive patient – with two nurses*

(a)

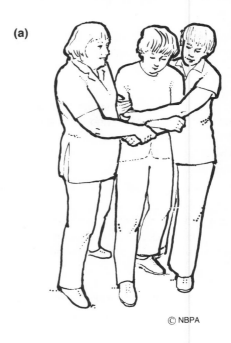

© NBPA

Fig 90b *Going down with patient to the floor as he falls*

(b)

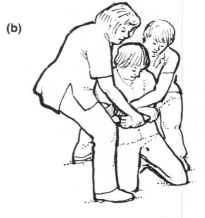

© NBPA

Whenever the patient lies on the floor out of choice (as distinct from falling) it is invariably safer to leave him where he is. If it is imperative to get him up again, the techniques described in Chapter 16, should be adopted.

When escorting an aggressive patient two nurses should hold the patients wrists, one on either side, with their other arms around the patient's waist (**Fig. 90a**). This will restrain the patient from striking out at the nurses. Should the patient fall, the nurses should then go down to the floor with him (**Fig. 90b**).

Whenever such patients need to be lifted bodily, control of the patient's upper and lower limbs is essential. The Through-arm Lift should be used in preference to any other in such cases, provided the patient is not too heavy, in which case a suitable sling and hoist should always be used.

The Backward Leaning Patient

The patient who has a tendency to lean backwards when being helped to his feet presents a common hazard to nurses. It is a neurological reaction triggered by fear and, like spasm, cannot be fought against; rather, a forward action should be encouraged by starting forward movements while the patient is still sitting in the chair and helping him to stand as a natural progression from this preparatory rocking. **The impetus must come from the patient, not from the nurse.** A 'heave' from the nurse will get a reflex pull backwards from the patient. Most dangerous of all is to allow such a patient to put his arms round the nurse's neck before he is up – he will literally suspend himself from her cervical spine. Time is well spent encouraging him to lean forward, and push up with his hands on the chair before allowing him to stand. It may be necessary to ask for help from a physiotherapist. Whether it be from nurse or physiotherapist, confident handling will help him to relax.

The Double-Leg Amputee Patient

If the patient is strong enough to use a sliding board, or transfer himself by using his arms, this is the best way. If he is not strong enough, a hoist with a one-piece hammock sling should be considered.

If the amputation is close to the knees, he may have to be lifted manually from bed to chair; the chair should be turned in towards the bed, and the patient sat on the edge of the bed with his back to the chair. The nurses can then put one knee on the bed, or sit on the bed, and lift him in two stages with either a Shoulder Lift (see Figure 50) or, depending on the relative heights of the patient and nurses, a Through-arm Lift with a handling sling. Figure 61 (Chapter 12) illustrates the first stage in this manoeuvre.

The Hemiplegic Patient

When planning the transfer of a hemiplegic patient, his specific needs must be considered:

- avoidance of any pressure on the affected shoulder joint

- blocking of the knee and foot on the affected side, which will prevent his knee from buckling and also enable him to lift his unaffected foot from the floor

- extra time taken in explanation, to ensure that he understands in which direction he is moving.

A handblock can often be used by the patient to move himself up the bed provided he has one good side. It enables him to raise his buttocks clear of the bed and he can then push down with his good leg to move up the bed. If he needs additional help, the nurse can use the Shoulder Lift on his weak side (**Fig. 91**). If he cannot get his affected shoulder across the nurse's back, she can hold it between her arm and chest. Either patient or the nurse can dictate the timing. The manoeuvre can be done in small steps. It should be practised before his discharge home.

Fig 91 *Use of handblocks by the patient*

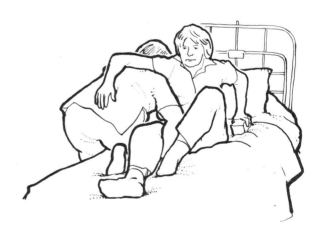

© NBPA

Nurses working in areas where hemiplegic patients are cared for will need special instruction from a physiotherapist.

Bobath Techniques for Hemiplegic Patients

Physiotherapists in specialised 'stroke' units sometimes teach the nurses how to use the Bobath technique (Bobath 1990) when transferring hemiplegic patients single-handed so that the rehabilitation process does not lapse when the patient is not receiving active therapy. The Bobath technique can indeed be helpful to patients and nurses alike when

Fig 92 *Use of the Charnley wedge*   **Fig 93** *Patient bridging*

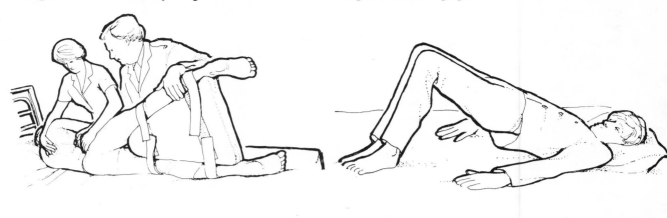

© NBPA   © NBPA

used for appropriately selected patients recovering from other disabling conditions. However, it is essentially therapeutic in nature, requiring a high level of training for the user, and should not be used by nurses unless they have received first hand instruction from a Bobath trained physiotherapist or other competent practitioner. Many nurses' injuries have occurred through using these techniques incorrectly for unsuitable patients.

Spasticity

Patients who go into spasm are always difficult to handle safely. It has been known for a nurse to be thrown across the room by a patient's violent spasm and as yet, nurses know little about how to control it. The following principles should be applied:

- Handle the patient firmly and avoid sudden movements.

- 'Fold him up' before attempting to move him. Extended positions predispose to spasm, flexed positions inhibit spasm.

- Encourage the patient to initiate movement; spasm commonly occurs as a reflex response to the nurse's movements.

- Preparatory movements such as rocking forward or thrusting the foot hard down onto the floor will inhibit spasm. Weight-bearing through the arm or leg also reduces it.

The Patient who Cannot Roll Unaided or Bridge

In some cases it is not medically possible to roll the patient, for example following hip surgery where rolling presents a risk. In these cases, a Charnley abduction wedge or two stout pillows can be used and the patient rolled safely onto the un-operated side (Love 1986) (**Fig. 92**).

However, there are also cases where the pelvis must be raised vertically in order to insert or remove a bed pan, change an incontinence pad or attend to pressure areas and the patient cannot help by pressing down with his hands and feet and raising his buttocks (**Fig. 93**). These procedures could last from several seconds to as many minutes. If a Pelvic Lift is performed by nurses unaided, they are not only exposed to the risks inherent in the Orthodox Lift, but those dangers are multiplied by the duration of the lift. Therefore, other methods must be found:

- A hoist (e.g. Mecanaids Ambulift Model D with an orthopaedic stretcher attachment);

- A divided mattress with a specially adapted bed that allows a section of the mattress under the buttocks to be lowered to give access;

- Where none of these methods are feasible, it may be possible to rig up a pulley/block system and raise the patient on hoist slings.

Chapter 18
Emergency Patient-handling Techniques and Methods of Evacuation

Introduction

In an emergency such as a fire, the safe and speedy evacuation of patients is a primary consideration. In these circumstances staff have to be particularly vigilant to observe the principles and rules of safe handling if they are to avoid injury. In hospitals and institutions for the care of the sick and elderly the authorities will have procedures for staff to follow in the emergency evacuation of the premises. These rules and procedures should be strictly followed*.

There are four basic methods of emergency evacuation. These are in order of priority; Walking, Wheeled transport, Sliding along the floor and Carrying.

Walking

Where patients and residents are able to walk they should be firmly told to walk to the assembly point. Some patients may have to be led to it. This should then leave the staff who are available to concentrate on those who cannot walk or who are bed-bound.

Wheeled Transport

Whenever possible it is invariably safer and less physically exhausting to evacuate a patient on

---

* A two part video presentation on Emergency Evacuation Techniques has been made. Part 1 Manual Techniques, Part 2 Mechanical Techniques. Enquiries to: Unit General Manager, Dudley Road Hospital, Dudley Road, Birmingham, B18 7QH.

wheeled equipment. Several items of equipment should be considered.

The bed makes a useful means of transport to evacuate the patient out of the immediate area of risk. However, this method has its limitations. The bed cannot travel other than on an even floor, and the bed or beds can create serious obstacles in corridors and at the top of stairs. The wheels need to be regularly maintained to ensure that they are free running. It is easier to pull rather than push the bed as this gives greater control.

Chairs fitted with wheels make an ideal means of transport. Equipment such as wheelchairs, commodes on wheels, sanichairs, and even easy chairs on castors can be pressed into service.

The Ambulance Carry Chair is compact both folded and opened, easily manoeuvrable, light to handle and rigid. It can be wheeled, but not lifted, by one person. There are several models available with either two or four small wheels.

The Carry Chair is, however, potentially unstable and should always be held by the handle at the back whenever a patient is sitting in it. A strap is provided to encircle the trunk and upper arms. This should be used to restrain the patient from grabbing at objects and pulling the chair over. The chair is designed to be tilted back when it is wheeled or carried. The patient should be warned of this.

The Carry Chair can be used to wheel or carry a patient downstairs. Two persons will be required if the chair is to be carried. When going downstairs, the

Fig 94 *Ambulance carry chair for use in emergencies*

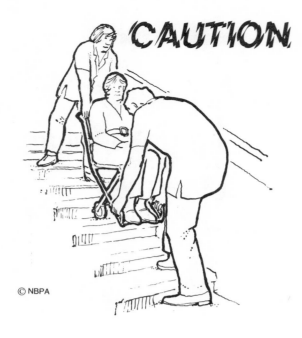

© NBPA

chair should be carried feet first with the nurse at the foot-end, walking backwards. The nurse holding the handle at the head-end should, if necessary, lean against the wall to help stabilise the lift and act as a brake. If a rest period is required, the chair should be put down on a stair tread as necessary but held constantly by the handle at the head-end (**Fig. 94**).

The Carry Chair should be used with extreme caution on stairs as the lifter at the foot end has to stoop.

The Quick-Evac Stretcher is a lightweight, low-cost stretcher, especially designed for the rapid evacuation of patients. It is made of a rigid pod-shaped shell of polyethylene, moulded so that the patient lies cocooned and strapped inside it. There are eight sets of small wheels along its underside which makes it easy for one person to pull across carpets. It can be taken downstairs provided sufficient help is available. Strong restraining straps are fitted at each end to enable the stretcher to be easily handled at floor level.

Sliding Along the Floor

Transferring a Patient Quickly to the Floor

The sliding method, which is for use by one or two persons is less stressful than lifting the patient. It is the preferred method whereby the patient lying in bed can be transferred to the floor quickly and safely in a controlled manner without the need to lift at all.

There is no need to lift a patient bodily from bed to floor. You can slide him.

- Place the bed at its lowest position, if height adjustable.

- Remove the bedclothes
- Slide the patient to the side of the bed nearest to you.
- Kneel by the side of the bed approximately in the middle on one knee.
- Ease the patient's body over the edge of the mattress ensuring that the patient's buttocks are lying on your raised thigh. Cradle the head and shoulders and gradually lower the patient to the floor.
- Once on the floor the patient can be rolled onto a sheet or blanket and pulled out on that, or by one of the methods described below.

It should be noted that for heavier patients, two persons kneeling by the side of the bed will be required.

Mattress, Ski Sheet and Ski Pad

The mattress on the bed provides a safe means of evacuation for the bed-bound patient. Its main advantage is that it can be dragged downstairs as well as along floors.

Some authorities provide specially made evacuation sheets which can be stored permanently under the mattress and used to even greater effect to achieve a mattress transfer.

The Ski Sheet is fitted with straps and lies permanently under the mattress. These may be found in high-dependency areas such as critical care. The straps can be easily pulled out from under the sides of the mattress. They are fastened together by a clunk click type car seat belt across the patient's trunk and legs. When pulled tight, the patient is held firmly on the mattress.

The bed should be put into its lowest position so that the mattress can then be eased off the bed onto the floor. The patient can then be pulled out of the area along floors and even downstairs. The mattress provides some protection for the patient from bumps and knocks.

This method is physically very demanding and preferably, two or more nurses should hold the lifting straps at the foot and head. It is not necessary however, to lift the mattress when pulling it along the floor.

The Ski Pad has been developed from the Ski Sheet and its main advantage is that it can negotiate narrow stairways, sharp bends, and narrow, twisting corridors with greater ease than a conventional bed mattress.

The Ski Pad is usually wall mounted in a ward in its own bag. The Ski Pad is laid on the floor and unfolded alongside the patient's bed. The patient is then transferred from the bed onto the Ski Pad (using the method of manual handling from mattress to floor) and wrapped in a blanket. The straps are fastened and the patient can then be pulled along the floor on its vinyl base. This pad will protect the patient from knocks and bruises.

Easy or dining chairs without wheels, may also be dragged backwards with a patient sitting in them.

Carrying

There is a wide variety of stretchers available although these may not normally be kept in patient areas. Carrying a stretcher is a physically demanding task over any distance and the following precautions are advised and should be observed whenever possible:

- Four persons should carry the stretcher one at each handle.
- The stronger persons should lift the stretcher at its head end.
- Twisting or rotation of the spine when loading manoeuvring or carrying a stretcher should be strictly avoided.
- One person must take control and give clear commands.
- If sufficient staff are not available to lift a stretcher in safety, other means of evacuation must be considered.

Manual techniques for emergency evacuation are methods of last resort. They are extremely stressful and exhausting. However in an emergency their use may be unavoidable.

Handling Principles

When speed is of the essence, the nurse is at greater risk of injury because there is no opportunity for recovery and the handling task cannot readily be pre-planned. This is the time when the normal principles of manual handling may be forgotten or disregarded because of imminent danger. For these reasons, nurses and other hospital workers are advised to plan ahead and practice these techniques using both equipment and manual methods so that should the situation arise, they are prepared.

For the purpose of the fire drill, all staff and particularly non-nursing staff should be given plenty of time to practice manual techniques under supervision, before being required to use the techniques under pressure. Only lightweight models should be used.

Handling Principles to Keep in Mind

- Slide rather than lift the patient.
- Do not attempt to lift anyone heavier than yourself.
- Keep the patient at floor level whenever possible.

What is a Standard?

A Standard is a professionally agreed level of performance. It must be appropriate to the situation, observable, achievable, measurable and desirable.

Standards based on the DYSSY System have been widely developed in the United Kingdom based on the pioneering work of Dr Alison Kitson, at the Radcliffe Infirmary, Oxford.

Employers are urged to establish their own standards for the Handling of Patients. These should be based on criteria which can be agreed locally and which can be measured to see if they are being achieved.

Criteria are variable indicators of the Standard and are based on the following:

1. **Structure Criteria**
   These are items of service which need to exist to enable the system to function:

   Buildings
   Policies, Rules
   Equipment and Services.

2. **Process Criteria**
   These are the means whereby the Standards are delivered in carrying out the task.

   Assessment procedure
   Delivery of Care
   Interventions
   Tools or equipment used
   How resources are used
   Determining Competencies.

3. **Outcome Criteria**
   This is the measurable element to see if the Standard has been achieved.

   The expected result
   The desirable outcome which can be measured.

Below is an example of a Local Standard on Patient handling:

Topic: The Handling of Patients

Client Group: Dependent or Semi-dependent Patients

Standard Statement:
All dependent or semi-dependent patients will be moved and handled by staff in a way which ensures maximum safety for the staff and minimal discomfort for the patients.

Structure Criteria

1. There is a patient handling policy based on the Manual Handling Operations Regulations 1992, regularly reviewed and updated.

2. All staff who may be required to handle patients will have knowledge of this policy.

3. The following equipment in sufficient numbers is provided: hoists; adjustable height beds and couches; sliding and transfer aids.

4. Staff have training which is based on demonstrated and verified competence.

5. There is a handling co-ordinator in post.

Process Criteria

1. An assessment of all handling activity is undertaken.

2. A safe system of handling for each patient will be agreed.

3. All reported back injuries will be fully investigated.

4. Staff will be assessed for their fitness to undertake manual handling.

5. Safeguards will be in place to protect staff when working in domestic premises.

Outcome Criteria

1. Patients are handled in safety, security and comfort.

2. Staff say they have less backache and are less tired.

3. Accident records of back injuries demonstrate a downward trend.

References

Anderson, J.A.D. & Sweetman, B.J. (1980). Heavy work and sickness-absence due to back pain. *Proceedings of British Association for Rheumatology and Rehabilitation*, Nottingham.

Baty, D., Stubbs, D.A., Buckle, P.W., Hudson, M.P. & Rivers, P.M. (1985). Working postures and associated stress in a nursing population. In: *Ergonomics International*, Eds I.D. Brown, R Goldsmith, K. Coombes, & M.A. Sinclair, pp 463-465. Taylor & Francis, London.

Biering-Sørensen, F. (1984). A prospective study of low back pain in a general population. I. Occurrence, recurrence and aetiology. *Scandinavian Journal of Rehabilitation Medicine*, **15**, 71-79.

Biering-Sørensen, F. (1984). Physical measurements as risk indicators for low back trouble over a one-year period. *Spine*, **9**, 106-119.

Bigos, S.J., Battié, M., Spengler, D.M., Fisher, L.D., Fordyce, W.E., Hansson, T., Nachemson, A.L. & Wortley, M.D. (1991). A prospective study of work perceptions and psychological factors affecting the report of back injury. *Spine*, **16**, 1-6.

Bobath, B. (1990). *Adult Hemiplegia: Evaluation and Treatment*. 3rd edition, Heinemann Medical Books, Oxford.

Brinckmann, P., Biggemann, M. & Hilweg, D. (1988). Fatigue fracture of human lumbar vertebrae. *Clinical Biomechanics*, Supplement 1.

Brinckmann, P., Biggemann, M. & Hilweg, D. (1989). Prediction of the compressive strength of human lumbar vertebrae. *Clinical Biomechanics*, Supplement 2.

BS 4467. (1991) *Dimensions in Designing for Elderly People*, British Standards Institution.

BS 5827. (1979). *Specification for Mobile Manually Operated Patient Lifting Devices*, British Standards Institution.

Chaffin, D.B., Herrin, G.D. & Keyserling, W.M. (1978). Pre-employment strength-testing: an updated position. *Journal of Occupational Medicine*, **20**, 403-408.

Chesterton, G.K. (1970). *The Wisdom of Father Brown*, Penguin, Harmondsworth.

Ciriello, V.M., Snook, S.H., Blick, A.C. & Wilkinson, P.L. (1990). The effects of task duration on psychophysically determined maximum acceptable weights and forces. *Ergonomics*, **33**, 187-200.

Commission of the European Communities. (1989a). *Council Directive on the Introduction of Measures to Encourage Improvements in the Safety and Health of Workers at Work*. **89/391/EEC**, Official Journal of the European Communities 29.6.89, No L 183/1-8, Brussels.

Commission of the European Communities. (1989b). *Council Directive Concerning the Minimum Safety and Health Requirements for the Use of Work Equipment by Workers at Work*. Second Individual Directive within the meaning of Article 16(1) of Directive 89/391/EEC, **89/655/EEC**, Official Journal of the European Communities 30.12.90, No L 393/13-17, Brussels.

Commission of the European Communities. (1990). *Council Directive on the Minimum Health and Safety Requirements for the Manual Handling of Loads where there is a Risk Particularly of Back Injury to Workers*. Fourth Individual Directive within the meaning of Article 16 (1) of Directive 89/391/EEC, **90/269/EEC**, Official Journal of the European Communities 21.6.90, No L 156/9-13, Brussels.

Corlett, E.N. (1990). Static muscle loading and the evaluation of posture. In: *Evaluation of Human Work: A Practical Ergonomics Methodology*, Eds. J.R.Wilson, & E.N. Corlett, pp 542-579. Taylor & Francis, London.

Corlett, E.N., Eklund, J.A.E., Reilly, T. & Troup, J.D.G. (1987). Assessment of workload from measurements of stature. *Applied Ergonomics*, **18**, 65-71.

Deyo, R.A., Diehl, A.K. & Rosenthal, M. (1986). How many days of bed rest for acute low back pain? *New England Journal of Medicine*, **315**, 1064-1070.

Dudley Road Hospital (1990). *Emergency Evacuation Techniques*, Video: Part 1– Manual Techniques, Part 2– Mechanical Techniques. Unit General Manager, Dudley Road Hospital, Dudley Road, Birmingham B18 7QH.

Eklund, J.A.E. & Corlett, E.N. (1984). Shrinkage as a measure of the effect of load on the spine. *Spine*, **9**, 189-194.

Farfan, H.F. (1977). A reorientation in the surgical approach to degenerative lumbar intervertebral joint disease. *Orthopaedic Clinics of North America*, **8**, 9-21.

Foreman, T.K. (1988). *Low back pain prevalence, work activity analysis and spinal shrinkage*. PhD Thesis, University of Liverpool.

Foreman, T.K., Davies, J.C. & Troup, J.D.G. (1988). A posture and activity classification system using a micro-computer. *International Journal of Industrial Ergonomics*, **2**, 285-289.

Foreman, T.K. & Troup, J.D.G. (1987). Diurnal variations in spinal loading and the effects of stature: a preliminary study of nursing activities. *Clinical Biomechanics*, **2**, 48-54.

Garg, A., Owen, B., Beller, D. & Banaag, J. (1991a). A biomechanical and ergonomic evaluation of patient transferring tasks: bed to wheelchair and wheelchair to bed. *Ergonomics*, **34**, 289-312.

Garg, A., Owen, B., Beller, D. & Banaag, J. (1991b). A biomechanical and ergonomic evaluation of patient transferring tasks: wheelchair to shower chair and shower chair to wheelchair. *Ergonomics*, **34**, 407-419.

Garg, A., Owen, B. & Carlson, B. (1992a). An ergonomic evaluation of nursing assistants' job in a nursing home. *Ergonomics*, **35**, 979-995.

Garg, A. & Owen, B. (1992b). Reducing back stress to nursing personnel: an ergonomic intervention in a nursing home. *Ergonomics*, **35**, 1353-1375.

Gilchrist, I.C. (1976). Psychiatric and social factors related to low back pain in general practice. *Rheumatology and Rehabilitation*, **15**, 101-107.

Goldsmith S., (1976). *Designing for the Disabled*. 3rd edition, RIBA Publications, London.

Green, W.H., & McCay, G.M. (1989). *Training Package for the Prevention of Back Injury*. Oxfordshire Health Authority.

Greenough, C.G. & Fraser, R.D. (1989). The effects of compensation on recovery from low-back injury. *Spine* **14**, 947-955.

Grieve, D.W. & Pheasant, S.T. (1981). Naturally preferred directions for the exertion of maximal manual forces. *Ergonomics* **24**, 684-693.

Harber, P., Billet, E., Shimozaki, S. & Vojtecky, M. (1988). Occupational back pain of nurses: special problems and prevention. *Applied Ergonomics*, **19**, 219-224.

Hayne, C., (1986). Evaluating the hazards of patient movement. *TalkBack*, **2**, **3**.

Health, Department of, (1986). *Common Activity Spaces*. Hospital Building Note, No 40, **1**, HMSO, London.

Health, Department of, (1989). *Discharge of Patients from Hospitals*. HC(89)5.

Health and Safety Commission. (1991a). *Proposals for Health and Safety (General Provisions) Regulations and Approved Code of Practice*. Consultative Document, CD34, Health and Safety Executive, London.

Health and Safety Commission. (1991b). *Provision and Use of Work Equipment: Draft Proposals for Regulations*. Consultative Document, CD35, Health and Safety Executive, London.

Health and Safety Commission. (1991c). *Manual Handling of Loads: Proposals for Regulation and Guidance*. Consultative Document, CD36, Health and Safety Executive, London.

Health and Safety Commission (1992a). *Management of health and safety at work*. Approved Code of Practice. HMSO, London.

Health and Safety Commission (1992b). *Workplace health, safety and welfare*. Approved Code of Practice. HMSO, London.

Health and Safety Executive (1992a). *Manual Handling*. Guidance on Regulations, L23, HMSO, London.

Health and Safety Executive (1992b). *Work equipment*. Guidance on Regulations, L22, HMSO, London.

Health Services Advisory Committee. (1984). *The Lifting of Patients in the Health Services*. Health & Safety Executive, HMSO, London.

Hirsch, C. (1955). The reaction of intervertebral discs to compression forces. *Journal of Bone & Joint Surgery*, **37-A**, 1188-1196.

Hollis, M. (1991). *Safer Lifting for Patient Care*. 3rd edition, Blackwell Scientific Publications, Oxford.

Hough, A. (1984). The effect of posture on lung function. *Physiotherapy*, **70**, 101-104.

Jensen, R.C. (1990). Back injuries among nursing personnel related to exposure. *Applied Occupational and Environmental Hygiene*, **5**, 38-45.

Jensen, R.C., Myers, A.H., Nestor, D., & Rattiner, J. (1988). *Low-back Injuries amongst Nursing Personnel: an Annotated Bibliography*. US Public Health Service, Division of Safety Research and The Johns Hopkins University, Injury Prevention Center, Baltimore.

Kazarian, L.E. (1972). Dynamic response characteristics of the human vertebral column. *Acta Orthopaedica Scandinavica*, Supplement 146.

Kazarian, L.E. (1975). Creep characteristics of the human spinal column. *Orthopaedic Clinics of North America*, **6**, 3-18.

Köller, W., Funke, F. & Hartman, F. (1981). Das Verformungsverhalten vom lumbalen menschlichen Zwishenwirbelscheiben unter langeinwirkender axialer dynamischer Druckkraft. *Zeitschrift für Orthopaedie und Ihre Grenzebiete* **119**, 206-216.

Lancet. (1965). The nurse's load. (Editorial). *Lancet*, 28th August 1965, **ii**, 422-423.

Ljungberg, A.-S., Kilbom, Å. & Hägg, G.M. (1989). Occasional lifting by nursing aides and warehouse workers. *Ergonomics*, **32**, 59-78.

Lloyd, S.G. & Breen, A.C. (1985). A study of back pain in nurses. *European Journal of Chiropractic*, **33**, 3-7.

Lloyd, D.C.E.F. & Troup, J.D.G. (1983). Recurrent back pain and its prediction. *Journal of the Society of Occupational Medicine*, **33**, 66-74.

Love, C. (1986). Do you roll or lift? *Nursing Times*, **82**, 44-46.

McAtamney L. & Corlett, E.N. (1992). Ergonomic workplace assessment in a healthcare context. *Ergonomics*, **35**, 965-978.

McCall, I.W., Park, W.M. & O'Brien, J.P. (1979). Induced pain referral from posterior elements in normal subjects. *Spine* **4**, 441-446.

Magnusson, M., Grandqvist, M., Jonson, R., Lindell, V., Lindberg, U., Wallin, L. & Hansson, T. (1990). The loads on the lumbar spine during work at an assembly line: the risks for fatigue injuries of vertebral bodies. *Spine*, **15**, 774-779.

Magora, A. (1970a). Investigation of the relationship between low back pain and occupation. Part I. Age, sex, community, education and other factors. *Industrial Medicine and Surgery of Trauma*, **39**, 465-471.

Magora, A. (1970b). Investigation of the relationship between low back pain and occupation. Part II. Work History. *Industrial Medicine and Surgery of Trauma*, **39**, 504-510.

Magora, A. (1972). Investigation of the relationship between low back pain and occupation. Part III. Physical requirements: sitting, standing and weight lifting. *Industrial Medicine and Surgery of Trauma*, **41**, 5-9.

Magora, A. (1973). Investigation of the relationship between low back pain and occupation. Part IV. Physical requirements: bending, rotation, reaching and sudden maximal effort. *Scandanavian Journal of Rehabilitation Medicine*, **5**, 186-190.

Management of Health and Safety at Work Regulations. (1992). *Statutory Instrument No 2051*, HMSO, London.

Manning, D.P., Mitchell, R.G. & Blanchfield, P.L. (1984). Body movements and events contributing to accidental and non-accidental back injuries. *Spine*, **9**, 734-739.

Manual Handling Operations Regulations. (1992). *Statutory Instrument No. 2793*, HMSO, London.

Moffett, J.A.K., Hughes, G.I. & Griffiths, P. (1992). A longitudinal study of back pain in student nurses. *International Journal of Nursing Studies*, paper accepted 1992.

Nurses, Midwives and Health Visitors Rules Approval Order. (1983). *Statutory Instrument No 873*, Rule 18, Training for admission to Parts 1-8 of the Register, pp 10-11, HMSO, London.

Osborne, C.M. (1978). *Low back pain in nurses*. BSc Dissertation, University of Surrey.

Owen, B.D. & Garg, A. (1989). Patient handling tasks perceived to be most stressful by nursing assistants. In: *Advances in Industrial Ergonomics and Safety I*, Ed. A.Mital, pp 775-781, Taylor & Francis, London.

Owen, B.D. & Garg, A. (1990). Assistive devices for use with patient handling tasks. In: *Advances in Industrial Ergonomics and Safety II*, Ed. B.Das, pp 585-792, Taylor & Francis, London.

Owen, B.D. & Garg, A. (1991) Reducing risk for back pain in nursing personnel. *American Association of Occupational Health Nurses Journal*, **39**, 24-32.

Perey, O. (1957). Fracture of the vertebral end-plate in the lumbar spine: an experimental biomechanical investigation. *Acta Orthopædica Scandinavica*, Supplement 25.

Pheasant, S. (1986). *Bodyspace: Anthropometry, Ergonomics and Design*. Taylor & Francis, London.

Pheasant, S. (1991). *Ergonomics, Work and Health*. Macmillan Academic and Professional, Basingstoke.

Pheasant, S. & Stubbs, D. (1992). Back pain in nurses: epidemiology and risk assessment. *Applied Ergonomics* 23, 226-232.

Porter, R.W., Hibbert, C. & Wellman, P. (1980). Backache and the lumbar spinal canal. *Spine*, 5, 99-105.

Provision and use of Work Equipment Regulations. (1992). *Statutory Instrument No. 2932*, HMSO, London.

Riihimäki, H. (1990). *Back disorders in relation to heavy physical work: a comparative study of concrete reinforcement workers and house painters*. Monograph (Doctoral Thesis), University of Helsinki, (ISBN 951 801 747 6).

Roaf, R. (1960). A study of the mechanics of spinal injuries. *Journal of Bone & Joint Surgery*, 42-B, 810-823.

Saari, J.(1987). Management of housekeeping by feedback. *Ergonomics*, 30, 313-317.

Sanchez, D. & Grieve, D.W. (1992). The measurement and prediction of isometric lifting strength in symmetrical and asymmetrical postures. *Ergonomics*, 35, 49-64.

Scholey, M. (1983). Back stress, the effects of training nurses to lift patients in a clinical situation. *International Journal of Nursing Studies*, 20, 1-13.

Sharp, G.R. (1985). *Occupationally Induced Back Pain in a Hospital Caring for Mentally Handicapped Patients*. Occupational Health Research Report, Forth Valley Health Board.

Snook, S.H. (1978). The design of manual handling tasks. *Ergonomics*, 21, 963-985.

Snook, S.H. & Ciriello, V.M. (1991). The design of manual handling tasks: Revised tables of maximum acceptable weights and forces. *Ergonomics*, 34, 1197-1213.

Stubbs, D.A., Buckle, P.W., Hudson, M.P., Rivers, P.M. & Worringham, C.J. (1983). Back pain in the nursing profession. I. Epidemiology and pilot methodology. *Ergonomics* 26, 755-765.

Takala, E.-P., Kukkonen, R. (1987). The handling of patients on geriatric wards. *Applied Ergonomics*, 18, 17-22.

Troup, J.D.G., Davies, J.C. & Manning, D.P. (1988). A model for the investigation of back injuries and manual handling problems at work. *Journal of Occupational Accidents*, 10, 107-119.

Troup, J.D.G. & Edwards, F.C. (1985) *Manual Handling and Lifting: An Information and Literature Review with Special Reference to the Back*. Health and Safety Executive, HMSO, London.

Troup, J.D.G., Foreman, T.K., Baxter, C.E. & Brown, D. (1987). The perception of back pain and the role of psychophysical tests of lifting capacity. *Spine*, 12, 645-657.

Troup, J.D.G., & Rauhala, H.H. (1987). Ergonomics and training. *International Journal of Nursing Studies*, 24, 325-330.

Troup, J.D.G. & Videman, T. (1989). Inactivity and the aetiopathogenesis of musculoskeletal disorders. Clinical *Biomechanics*, 4, 173-178.

Tyrrell, A.R., Reilly, T. & Troup, J.D.G. (1985). Circadian variation in stature and the effects of spinal loading. *Spine*, 10, 161-164.

Vasey, J. & Crozier, L. (1982). A neuromuscular approach to handling and lifting. *Nursing Mirror*, Issues April 28, May 5,12,19,26, June 2.

Venning, P.J., Walter, S.D. & Stitt, L.W. (1987). Personal and job-related factors as determinants of incidence of back injuries among nursing personnel. *Journal of Occupational Medicine*, 29, 820-825.

Versloot, J.M., Rozeman, A., Son, A.M. van., Akkerveeken, P.F. van. (1992). The cost effectiveness of a back school program in industry: a longitudinal controlled field study. *Spine*, 17, 22-27.

Videman, T., Nurminen, T., Tola, S., Kuorinka, I., Vanharanta H. & Troup, J.D.G. (1984). Low-back pain in nurses and some loading factors of work. *Spine*, 9, 400-404.

Videman, T., Rauhala, H., Lindström, K., Cedercreutz, G., Kämppi, M., Tola, S. & Troup, J.D.G. (1989). Patient-handling skill, back injuries, and back pain: an intervention study in nursing. *Spine*, 14, 148-156.

Waddell, G., Main, C.G., Morris, E.W., Paola, M. di, & Gray, I.C.M. (1984). Chronic low back pain: psychologic distress and illness behavior. *Spine*, 9, 209-213.

Williams J.P.R. & McKibbin, B. (1978). Cervical spine injuries in Rugby Union football. *British Medical Journal*, ii, 1747.

Wilson J.R. & Corlett, E.N. (1990). (Editors). *Evaluation of Human Work: A Practical Ergonomics Methodology*. Taylor & Francis, London.

Workplace (Health, Safety and Welfare) Regulations. (1992). *Statutory Instrument No. 3004*, HMSO, London.

Wyke, B.(1976). Neurological aspects of low back pain. In: *The Lumbar Spine and Back Pain*, Ed. M.I.V. Jayson, pp 189-256. Sector Publishing, London.

Disabled Living Centres

ABERDEEN
Hillylands Disabled Centre,
Croft Road,
Mastrick,
Aberdeen, AB2 6RB.
0224 685247

AYLESBURY
Stoke Mandeville Independent Living Exhibition,
Stoke Mandeville Hospital,
Mandeville Road,
Aylesbury,
Bucks, HP21 8AL.
0296 84111 x 3114

BELFAST
Disabled Living Centre, Regional Disablement Services,
Musgrave Park Hospital,
Stockman's Lane,
Belfast, B19 7JB.
0232 669501 x 2708

BIRMINGHAM
Disabled Living Centre,
260 Broad Street,
Birmingham, B1 2HF.
021 643 0980

BODELWYDDAN
North Wales Resource Centre for Disabled People,
Ysbyty Glan Clwyd,
Bodelwyddan,
Clywd, LL18 5UJ.
0745 583910 x 4706/4609

BRAINTREE
Independent Living Advice Centre,
Black Notley Hospital,
Braintree,
Essex.
0376 21068

CAERPHILLY
Resources (Aids & Equipment) Centre,
Wales Council for the Disabled,
"Llys Ifor", Crescent Road,
Caerphilly,
Mid-Glamorgan, CF8 1XL.
0222 887325/6/7

CARDIFF
Disabled Living Centre,
The Lodge,
Rockwood Hospital,
Fairwater Road Liandaff,
Cardiff,
South Glamorgan
0222 566281 x 3751

COLCHESTER
Disabled Living Centre,
Occupational Therapy Depart,
Colchester General Hosp,
Colchester,
0206 853535 x 2172/2173

EDINBURGH
Lothian Disabled Living Centre,
Astley Ainslie Hospital,
Grange Loan,
Edinburgh, EH9 2HL.
031 447 6271 x 5635

EXETER
Independent Living Centre,
St Loye's School of Occupational Therapy,
Millbrook House,
Topsham Road,
Exeter, EX2 6ES.
0392 59260

HUDDERSFIELD
Disabled Living Centre,
Kirklees Social Services,
Unit 6, Silvercourt Trading Estate,
Silver Street,
Huddersfield,
West Yorks.
0484 518809

HULL
St Hilda House,
National Demonstration Centre,
Kingston General Hospital,
Beverley Road,
Hull, HU3 1UR.
0482 28631 x 332

INVERNESS
Disabled Living Centre,
Raigmore Hospital,
Inverness, IV2 3UJ.
0463 234151 x 293

MIDDLESBROUGH
Department of Rehabilitation,
Middlesbrough General Hospital,
Ayresome Green Lane,
Middlesbrough,
Cleveland, TS5 5AZ.
0642 850222 x 158

LEEDS
The William Merritt Disabled Living Centre,
St Mary's Hospital,
Greenhill Road,
Leeds, LS12 3QE.
0532 793140

LEICESTER
The Disabled Living Centre,
Red Cross Medical Aid Dept,
76 Clarendon Park Road,
Leicester,
LE2 3AD.
0533 700747

LIVERPOOL
Merseyside Centre for Independent Living,
Youens Way,
East Prescot Road,
Liverpool.
051 228 9221

LONDON
The Disabled Living Foundation,
380/384 Harrow Road,
London,
W9 2HU.
071 289 6111

MAC (MOBILE ADVICE CENTRE)
A Mobile Exhibition Touring Scotland,
Details from:
Disability Scotland,
Princes House,
5 Shandwick Place,
Edinburgh, EH2 4RG.
031 229 8632

MACCLESFIELD
Disabled Living Centre,
Macclesfield District General Hospital,
Victoria Road,
Macclesfield,
Cheshire, SK10 3BL.
0625 6621740

MANCHESTER
Regional Disabled Living Centre,
Disabled Living Services,
Redbank House,
4 St Chad's Street,
Cheetham,
Manchester.
061 832 3678

NEWCASTLE upon TYNE
Newcastle upon Tyne Council for the Disabled,
The Dene Centre,
Castles Farm Road,
Newcastle upon Tyne.
091 284 0480

NOTTINGHAM
Nottingham Resource Centre for the Disabled,
Lenton Business Centre,
Lenton Boulevard,
Nottingham, NG7 2BY.
0602 420391

PAISLEY
Disability Centre for Independent Living,
Community Services Centre,
Queen Street,
Paisley,
Strathclyde.
041 887 0597

PORTSMOUTH
The Frank Sorrell Centre,
Prince Albert Road,
Eastney,
Portsmouth, PO4 4HR.
0705 737174

SEMINGTON
Western Wiltshire Disabled Living Centre,
St George's Hospital,
Semington,
Wiltshire, BA14 6JQ.
0380 871007

SOUTHAMPTON
Southampton Aid & Equipment Centre,
Southampton General Hosp,
Tremona Road,
Southampton, SO9 4XY.
0703 796631

STOCKPORT
Disabled Living Centre,
St Thomas' Hospital,
Shawheath,
Stockport,
Cheshire.
061 419 4476

SWANSEA
Disabled Living Assessment Centre,
St John's Road,
Manselton,
Swansea, SA5 8PR.
0792 580161

SWINDON
The Swindon Centre for Disabled Living,
The Hawthorne Centre,
Cricklade Road,
Swindon,
Wiltshire.
0793 643966

WELWYN GARDEN CITY
Easier Living Exhibition,
Hertfordshire,
Association for the Disabled,
The Woodside Centre,
The Commons,
Welwyn Garden City,
Herts.
0707 324581

For further information contact:
Disabled Living Centre's Council
286 Camden Road
London
N7 OBJ
071 700 1707

Index

Notes